P9-DCI-729

SOLUTIONS TO THE EXERCISES IN

Principles of

Imaging Science and Protection

Michael A. Thompson, M.S.
Professor, Medical Physics
Division of Medical Imaging and Therapy
The University of Alabama at Birmingham
Birmingham, Alabama

Janice D. Hall, M.A. Ed., R.T.(R.)
Assistant Professor and Director
Advanced Imaging Program
The University of Alabama at Birmingham
Birmingham, Alabama

Marian P. Hattaway, B.S., R.T.(R.)
Associate Professor
Radiography Program
The University of Alabama at Birmingham
Birmingham, Alabama

Steven B. Dowd, Ed. D., R.T.(R.)
Program Director
Assistant Professor
Radiography Program
The University of Alabama at Birmingham
Birmingham, Alabama

W.B. SAUNDERS COMPANY
A Division of Harcourt Brace & Company
Philadelphia London Toronto Montreal Sydney Tokyo

W. B. SAUNDERS COMPANY
A Division of
Harcourt Brace & Company

The Curtis Center
Independence Square West
Philadelphia, Pennsylvania 19106

Solutions to the Exercises in
PRINCIPLES OF IMAGING SCIENCE AND PROTECTION   0-7216-3430-3

Printed in the United States of America

Last digit is the print number: 9   8   7   6   5   4   3   2   1

TABLE OF CONTENTS

I. TEXT SOLUTIONS

Chapter 1 . . . . page 1

Chapter 2 . . . . page 3

Chapter 3 . . . . page 17

Chapter 4 . . . . page 25

Chapter 5 . . . . page 34

Chapter 6 . . . . page 42

Chapter 7 . . . . page 47

Chapter 8 . . . . page 58

Chapter 9 . . . . page 66

Chapter 10 . . . . page 71

Chapter 11 . . . . page 72

Chapter 12 . . . . page 90

Chapter 13 . . . . page 94

Chapter 14 . . . . page 117

Chapter 15 . . . . page 119

Chapter 16 . . . . page 122

Chapter 17 . . . . page 123

Chapter 18 . . . . page 125

Chapter 19 . . . . page 128

Chapter 20 . . . . page 131

Chapter 21 . . . . page 137

Chapter 22 . . . . page 141

II. Workbook Solutions

Worksheet 2-1 . . . . page 143

Worksheet 2-2 . . . . page 146

Worksheet 2-3 . . . . page 147

Worksheet 2-4 . . . . page 149

Worksheet 2-5 . . . . page 153

Worksheet 2-6 . . . . page 155

Worksheet 2-7 . . . . page 157

Worksheet 2-8 . . . . page 161

Worksheet 2-9 . . . . page 164

Worksheet 2-10 . . . . page 167

Worksheet 2-11 . . . . page 169

Worksheet 2-12 . . . . page 169

Worksheet 3-1 . . . . page 170

Worksheet 3-2 . . . . page 171

Worksheet 3-3 . . . . page 171

Worksheet 3-4 . . . . page 173

Worksheet 3-5 . . . . page 175

Worksheet 4-1 . . . . page 176

Worksheet 4-2 . . . . page 177

Worksheet 4-3 . . . . page 179

Worksheet 4-4 . . . . page 182

Worksheet 5-1 . . . . page 183

Worksheet 5-2 . . . . page 184

Worksheet 6-1 . . . . page 187

Worksheet 7-1 . . . . page 188

Worksheet 8-1 . . . . page 189

Worksheet 8-2 . . . . page 190

Worksheet 10-1 . . . . page 193

Worksheet 15-1 . . . . page 194

Worksheet 16-1 . . . . page 194

Worksheet 17-1 . . . . page 195

Worksheet 18-1 . . . . page 195

Worksheet 18-2 . . . . page 196

Worksheet 19-1 . . . . page 196

Worksheet 21-1 . . . . page 197

CHAPTER 1 SOLUTIONS

1. X-ray photons are packets of pure electromagnetic energy like light but much more penetrating. They carry zero mass and zero electric charge.

2. In an x-ray tube, electrons emitted from the filament are accelerated from the negatively charged cathode to the positively charged anode. The great increase in electron speed results from the high voltage placed across the tube electrodes. The fast moving electrons strike the tungsten target where their energy is converted into heat (~99%) and
    x-rays (~1%).

3. The filament, when heated, becomes the source of the electrons needed for x-ray production.

    The cathode, being the negative electrode, repels the electrons emitted from the filament toward the positively charged anode.

    A target having a high Z-number and a high melting point (e.g., tungsten) is the material with which the fast moving electrons interact to produce x-rays.

    The anode is the positive electrode of the x-ray tube and attracts the negatively charged electrons into the tube target.

    The glass envelope provides mechanical support for the x-ray tube components and maintains the vacuum conditions within the tube.

    The high voltage generator provides the high voltage which is necessary to accelerate the electrons into the target.

4   a. The greater the number of electrons flowing between the x-ray

tube electrodes (i.e., the tube current), the greater the number of x-rays produced.

    b. The greater the voltage placed across the x-ray tube electrodes, the more energetic or more penetrating the x-rays produced.

5. An x-ray photon striking a patient's body may interact with the tissue it encounters by:

    a. transmission through the tissue with no change in its original direction of travel, resulting in a dark area on the radiographic film, or

    b. absorption within the tissue, resulting in a light area on the radiograph, or

    c. scattering within the tissue, resulting in shades of gray on the radiograph.

6. Scatter radiation contributes to film fog, which only degrades the diagnostic quality of the radiograph.

7. Two sources of scatter radiation are the patient and the imaging table top.

8. Time, distance, and appropriate shielding.

9. The radiographer can reduce radiation exposure to the patient by using (1) the correct technical factors to reduce the need for repeat films, (2) proper beam collimation, and (3) gonadal shielding.

10. Film badge readings should accurately represent only the radiation dose received by the individual. If the badge receives additional radiation exposure while it is in storage, this results in an erroneously high radiation dose ascribed to the individual.

CHAPTER 2   SOLUTIONS

1. a. $\dfrac{1}{3} + \dfrac{1}{4} = \dfrac{4}{12} + \dfrac{3}{12} = \dfrac{7}{1}$

   b. $\dfrac{2}{3} + \dfrac{1}{5} = \dfrac{10}{15} + \dfrac{3}{15} = \dfrac{13}{15}$

   c. $\dfrac{2}{3} \times \dfrac{1}{4} = \dfrac{2 \times 1}{3 \times 4} = \dfrac{2}{12} = \dfrac{1}{6}$

   d. $\dfrac{1}{5} \times \dfrac{5}{7} = \dfrac{1 \times 5}{5 \times 7} = \dfrac{1}{7}$

   e. $\dfrac{1}{3} \div \dfrac{1}{5} = \dfrac{1}{3} \times \dfrac{5}{1} = \dfrac{5}{3}$

   f. $2 \div \dfrac{2}{3} = \dfrac{2}{1} \times \dfrac{3}{2} = 3$

2. a. $\dfrac{3}{5} = \dfrac{x}{6}$

      $5x = 18$

      $x = \dfrac{18}{5}$

   b. $\dfrac{1}{4} = \dfrac{2}{x}$

      $(1)(x) = (2)(4)$

      $x = 8$

   c. $\dfrac{5}{6} = \dfrac{x}{4}$

      $(6)x = (5)(4)$

      $6x = 20$

      $x = \dfrac{20}{6} \; or \; \dfrac{10}{3}$

d.
$$\frac{x}{3} = \frac{8}{7}$$
$$(7)(x) = (3)(8)$$
$$7x = 24$$
$$x = \frac{24}{7}$$

3. a. $\frac{1}{4} = 1 \div 4 = 0.25$

    b. $\frac{2}{3} = 2 \div 3 \approx 0.67$

    c. $\frac{2}{5} = 2 \div 5 = 0.4$

    d. $\frac{1}{10} = 1 \div 10 = 0.1$

4. a. $0.25 = \frac{25}{100} = \frac{1}{4}$

    b. $0.60 = \frac{60}{100} = \frac{6}{10} = \frac{3}{5}$

    c. $0.125 = \frac{125}{1000} = \frac{5}{40} = \frac{1}{8}$

    d. $0.2 = \frac{2}{10} = \frac{1}{5}$

5. a. $2^5 = 32$

    b. $e^3 = (2.718)^3 \approx 20.08$

    c. $\log 150 \approx 2.18$

    d. $\ln 28 \approx 3.3$

    e. $\log 1 = 0$

6. a. positive exponential
    b. linear (direct)
    c. negative exponential
    d. linear (indirect)

7. a. $25600 = 2.56 \times 10^4$

4

b. 1.00   = 1.00 x 10^0

c. 0.00323 = 3.23 x 10^{-3}

d. 0.000012 = 1.2 x 10^{-5}

e. 4153 = 4.153 x 10^3

8. a. 2400 x 0.0002 = (2.4 x 10^3)(2 x 10^{-4})

$\qquad\qquad\qquad$ = 4.8 x 10^{-1}

b. 0.0006 x 0.002 x 0.00005 = (6 x 10^{-4})(2 x 10^{-3})(5 x 10^{-5})

$\qquad\qquad\qquad\qquad\qquad$ = 60 x 10^{-12}

$\qquad\qquad\qquad\qquad\qquad$ = 6 x 10^{-11}

c. 25 x 2000 x 0.002 = (2.5 x 10^1)(2 x 10^3)(2 x 10^{-3})

$\qquad\qquad\qquad\qquad$ = 10 x 10^1 = 10^2

d. (2 x 10^3)^2 = 4 x 10^6

e. $\dfrac{80,000}{0.004} = \dfrac{8 \times 10^4}{4 \times 10^{-3}} = 2 \times 10^7$

f. $\dfrac{0.0006}{400} = \dfrac{6 \times 10^{-4}}{4 \times 10^2} = \dfrac{3}{2} \times 10^{-6} = 1.5 \times 10^{-6}$

9. a. Convert 10 cm to inches:

$10 \text{ cm} \times \dfrac{1 \text{ in}}{2.54 \text{ cm}} \approx 3.9 \text{ in}$

b. Convert 120 lbs to kg:

$120 \text{ lbs} \times \dfrac{1 \text{ kg}}{2.2 \text{ lbs}} = 54.5 \text{ kg}$

c. Convert 10 inches to mm:

$10 \text{ in} \times \dfrac{2.54 \text{ cm}}{1 \text{ in}} \times \dfrac{10 \text{ mm}}{1 \text{ cm}} = 254 \text{ mm}$

d. Convert 2 hrs to ms:

$2 \text{ } hrs \times \dfrac{60 \text{ min}}{1 \text{ } hr} \times \dfrac{60 \text{ } s}{1 \text{ min}} \times \dfrac{10^3 ms}{1 \text{ } s} = 7.2 \times 10^6 ms$

e. Convert 50 kg to lbs:

$50 \text{ } kg \times \dfrac{2.2 \text{ } lbs}{1 \text{ } kg} = 110 \text{ } lbs$

f. Convert 5 m to μm:

$$5\ m \times \frac{10^6 \mu m}{1\ m} = 5 \times 10^6 \mu m$$

g. Convert 10 km to cm:

$$10\ km \times \frac{10^3 m}{1\ km} \times \frac{10^2\ cm}{1\ m} = 10^6\ cm.$$

10. $$v = \frac{d}{t} = \frac{15\ m}{0.5\ s} = 30\ \frac{m}{s}$$

11. $$v = \frac{d}{t} = \frac{40\ m}{10\ ms} = \frac{40\ m}{10 \times 10^{-3} s} = \frac{40 m}{10^{-2} s} = 4 \times 10^3 \frac{m}{s}$$

12. $$a = \frac{v}{t} = \frac{50\frac{m}{s} - 10\frac{m}{s}}{0.1\ s} = \frac{40\ \frac{m}{s}}{1 \times 10^{-1} s} = 4 \times 10^2\ \frac{m}{s^2}$$

13. It can change its direction of motion.

14. A net force must be applied to a body to produce an acceleration.

15. "Net" force implies an unbalanced force - that is, the force which remains when all forces acting on a body are added together taking into account their magnitude (size) and direction.

16. It causes the body to undergo an acceleration, i.e., it causes the object to increase its speed, decrease its speed, or change its direction of motion.

17. Direct relationship; direct relationship.

18. More difficult.

19. p = mv

= (10 kg)(20 m/s)

= 200 kg-m/s

20. $KE = 1/2 \ mv^2$

$= 1/2 (5 \ kg)(10 \ m/s)^2$

$= 1/2 (5 \ kg)(100 \ m^2/s^2)$

$= 250$ joules　　　　　**NOTE:** 1 joule = 1 kg-m^2/s^2

21. $KE = 1/2 \ mv^2$

$= 1/2 (0.1 \ kg)(4 \ m/s)^2$

$= 1/2 (0.1 \ kg)(16 \ m^2/s^2)$

$= 0.8$ joules　　　　　**NOTE:** gms must be converted to kg, the SI

unit of mass

22. Direct relationship; direct relationship.

23.
$$1.6 \times 10^{-14} \, joules \times \frac{1 \ eV}{1.6 \times 10^{-19} \, joules} = 10^5 \ eV;$$

$$10^5 \ eV \times \frac{1 \ keV}{10^3 \ eV} = 10^2 \ keV \ or \ 100 \ keV$$

24. $E = mc2$

$= (10^{-3} \ kg)(3 \times 10^8 \ m/s)^2$

$= (10^{-3} \ kg)(9 \times 10^{16} \ m^2/s^2)$

$= 9 \times 10^{13}$ joules　　　**NOTE:** gms must again be converted to kg.

25. a. converts electrical energy to heat energy

b. converts electrical energy to sound energy

c. converts electrical energy to light energy

d. converts light (or sound) into electrical (or mechanical)

energy

26. $P = E/t$

$= 50 \ J/0.5 \ s$

$= 100$ watts　　　　　**NOTE:** 1 watt = 1 joule/second

27. P = E/t   or

     E = P x t

        = (2000 watts)(1 min)   **NOTE:** minutes must be converted to

        = (2000 J/s)(60 s)   seconds to get units energy

        = 1.2 x 10⁵ J   (i.e., joules)

28. $P = \dfrac{E}{t}$

    $= \dfrac{100 \; J}{0.25 \; s}$

    $= 400 \; watts$

29. Since heat is energy, it can be measured in the SI unit of
     energy, the joule.

30. a. convection - heat transfer by a fluid (here, blood)

     b. conduction - primary mode of heat transfer in metals

     c. convection - heat transfer by a fluid (here, air)

     d. radiation - body gives off visible radiation

31. a. $T_c = 5/9 (T_F - 32°)$

            $= 5/9 (10° - 32°)$

            $= 5/9 (-22°)$

            $= -12.2°C$

     b. $T_F = 9/5 \; T_c + 32°$

            $= 9/5 (50°) + 32°$

            $= 90° + 32°$

            $= 122° \; F$

     c. $T_F = 9/5 \; T_c + 32°$

            $= 9/5 (-100°) + 32°$

            $= -180° + 32°$

            $= -148°F$

d. $T_c = 5/9(T_F - 32°)$

$\qquad = 5/9(0 - 32°)$

$\qquad \approx -17.8° \text{ C}$

EXERCISE SOLUTIONS

1. a. $(3 \times 10^{-2})^2(2 \times 10^4)^3 = (9 \times 10^{-4})(8 \times 10^{12})$

$\qquad\qquad\qquad\qquad = 72 \times 10^8 = 7.2 \times 10^9$

 b. $(100)°(2 \times 10^6)^3 = (1)(8 \times 10^{18}) = 8 \times 10^{18}$

 c. $\dfrac{(2 \times 10^5)(5 \times 10^1)}{(200)^3} = \dfrac{10 \times 10^6}{(2 \times 10^2)^3} = \dfrac{1 \times 10^7}{8 \times 10^6}$

$\qquad\qquad\qquad = 0.125 \times 10^1$

$\qquad\qquad\qquad = 1.25$

 d. $(\sqrt{400})(10^6)^{-2} = (20)(10^{-12}) = 2 \times 10^{-11}$

2. a. $\dfrac{1}{x} = \dfrac{1}{3} + \dfrac{1}{4}$

$\qquad = \dfrac{4}{12} + \dfrac{3}{12}$

$\qquad = \dfrac{7}{12}$

$\quad x = \dfrac{12}{7}$

9

b. $\dfrac{1}{2} = \dfrac{1}{x} + \dfrac{1}{5}$

$\dfrac{1}{x} = \dfrac{1}{2} - \dfrac{1}{5}$

$\phantom{\dfrac{1}{x}} = \dfrac{5}{10} - \dfrac{2}{10}$

$\phantom{\dfrac{1}{x}} = \dfrac{3}{10}$

$x = \dfrac{10}{3}$

c. $\qquad \dfrac{10\ in}{x} = \dfrac{1\ in}{2.54\ cm}$

$(1\ in)(x) = (2.54\ cm)(10\ in)$

$x = 25.4\ cm$

d. $\qquad \dfrac{20\ kg}{x} = \dfrac{1\ kg}{2.2\ lbs}$

$(x)(1\ kg) = (20\ kg)(2.2\ lbs)$

$x = 44\ lbs$

e. $\qquad \dfrac{x}{5\ min} = \dfrac{6 \times 10^4\ ms}{1\ min}$

$(x)(1\ min) = (5\ min)(6 \times 10^4\ ms)$

$x = 3 \times 10^5\ ms$

3. a. Convert 10 oz to mg:

$$10\ oz \times \dfrac{1\ lb}{16\ oz} \times \dfrac{1\ kg}{2.2\ lbs} \times \dfrac{10^3 gm}{1\ kg} \times \dfrac{10^3 mg}{1\ gm} \approx 2.8 \times 10^5\ mg$$

b. Convert 1/4 lb to μgm:

$$0.25\ lb \times \dfrac{1\ kg}{2.2\ lbs} \times \dfrac{10^3 gm}{1\ kg} \times \dfrac{10^6 \mu gm}{1\ gm} \approx 1.14 \times 10^8\ \mu gm$$

c. Convert 10 m² to ft²:

$$\approx 107.7 \ ft^2$$

d. Convert 100 cc to in³:

$$10^2 \ cm^3 \times \left(\frac{1 \ in}{2.54 \ cm}\right)^3 \approx 10^2 \ cm^3 \times \frac{1 \ in^3}{16.39 \ cm^3} \approx 6.1 \ in^3$$

NOTES: 1. It should be pointed out to students that each factor used in the dimensional analysis technique has a numerical value of 1. Thus squaring or cubing these factors has no effect

(i.e., $1^2 = 1^3 = 1$) except on unit cancellation.

2. When using pocket calculators, a common mistake students make is to enter powers such as 10^6 by entering "10" then "EXP(ONENT)6." It should be pointed out that when entering powers of 10 with the exponent key, one enters "1" then "EXP 6." If 10 is first entered, the answer will be off by a factor of 10.

e. Convert 10^{20} µs to days:

$$10^{20}\mu s \times \frac{1 \ s}{10^6 \mu s} \times \frac{1 \ min}{60 \ s} \times \frac{1 \ hr}{60 \ min} \times \frac{1 \ day}{24 \ hr} \approx 1.16 \times 10^9 \ days$$

f. Convert 10 ft³ to mm³:

$$10 \ ft^3 \times \left(\frac{12 \ in}{1 \ ft}\right)^3 \times \left(\frac{2.54 \ cm}{1 \ in}\right)^3 \times \left(\frac{10 \ mm}{1 \ cm}\right)^3$$

$$= 10 \ ft^3 \times \frac{1728 \ in^3}{1 \ ft^3} \times \frac{16.39 \ cm^3}{1 \ in^3} \times \frac{10^3 \ mm^3}{1 \ cm^3}$$

$$= 2.8 \times 10^8 \ mm^3$$

4. a. $\log 250 \approx 2.398$

   b. $\ln 250 \approx 5.521$

   c. $\ln 1 = 0$

   d. $\log 1 = 0$

   e. $x = e^{2.5} \approx 12.18$

   f. $x = 10^{2.5} \approx 316.23$

   g. $5 e^x = 25$

   $e^x = 5$

   $\ln (e^x) = \ln 5$

   $x(1) = 1.609$

   $x = 1.609$

   h. $10 e^x = 45$

   $e^x = 4.5$

   $\ln (e^x) = \ln (4.5)$

   $x(1) = 1.504$

   $x = 1.504$

   i. $\log_{10} x = 1.8$

   Using the definition of a logarithm, this can be rewritten in the form:

   $$10^{1.8} = x$$

   or

   $$x \approx 63.1$$

   j. $\ln_e x = 2.1$

   Again using the definition of a logarithm, the equation can be rewritten as:

   $$e^{2.1} = x$$

   or

   $$x \approx 8.17$$

k. $10(0.5)^x = 2$

$(0.5)^x = 0.2$

$\ln(0.5)^x = \ln(0.2)$ or

$x\ln(0.5) = \ln(0.2)$

$x(-0.693) = -1.609$

$x \approx 2.32$

$10(0.5)^x = 2$

$(0.5)^x = 0.2$

$\log(0.5)^x = \log(0.2)$

$x\log(0.5) = \log(0.2)$

$x(-0.301) = (-0.699)$

$x \approx 2.32$

NOTE: In this case, since the base number is 0.5, it does not matter which logarithm is used. One obtains the same answer by either method.

l. $4(0.5)^x = 0.6$

$(0.5)^x = 0.15$

$\ln(0.5)_x = \ln(0.15)$ or

$x\ln(0.5) = \ln(0.15)$

$x(-0.693) = (-1.897)$

$x \approx 2.74$

$4(0.5)^x = 0.6$

$(0.5)^x = 0.15$

$\log(0.5)^x = \log(0.15)$

$x\log(0.5) = \log(0.15)$

$x(-0.301) = (-0.824)$

$x \approx 2.74$

5. a. $y = 45$ when $x = 45$

   b. $x = 24$ when $y = 64$

   c. $y \approx 32$ when $x = 3.5$

   d. $y = 1$ when $x = 0$; This is verified because $y = e^0 = 1$

   e. $y = 1$ when $x = 0$; This is also verified because

      $y = e^{-0} = 1$

   f. y varies indirectly with x since y decreases as x

      increases.

   g. $y \approx 0.6$ when $x = 0.5$; $y \approx 0.082$ when $x = 2.5$;

      $y = 0.003$ when $x = 5.8$; $y = 0.0015$ when $x = 6.5$

   h. 5 powers of 10 are represented (i.e., 10^{-3}, 10^{-2}. 10^{-1},

      10^0, 10^1)

6. Given: $v = 10^3$ m/s

   $t = 1$ min $= 60$ s

   $d = ?$

   $v = d/t$

   or $d = v \times t$

   $= (10^3$ m/s$)(60$ s$)$

   $= 6 \times 10^4$ m

   $(6 \times 10^4$ m$) \times \dfrac{10^2 \text{cm}}{1 \text{ m}} \times \dfrac{1 \text{ in}}{2.54 \text{ cm}} \times \dfrac{1 \text{ ft}}{12 \text{ in}} \times \dfrac{1 \text{ mile}}{5280 \text{ ft}}$

   ≈ 37.28 miles

7. Given: $v = 10^3$ m/s

   $d = 2$ in

   $t = ?$

   First convert 2 in to m so units will cancel:

   $$d = 2 \ in \times \frac{2.54 \ cm}{1 \ in} \times \frac{1 \ m}{10^2 \ cm} \approx 0.05 \ m$$

   Then solve the velocity equation for time (t):

   $$v = \frac{d}{t}$$

   $$t = \frac{d}{v}$$

   $$= \frac{0.05 \ m}{10^3 \frac{m}{s}}$$

   $$\approx 5 \times 10^{-5} \ s \ or \ 50 \mu s$$

8. Given: $\Delta v = 150$ m/s $- 10$ m/s

   $= 140$ m/s

   $\Delta t = 0.5$ min $= 30$ s

   $a = ?$

Using the definition of acceleration,

$$a = \frac{\Delta v}{\Delta t}$$

$$= 140\frac{\frac{m}{s}}{30\ s}$$

$$\approx 4.67\frac{m}{s^2}$$

9. Since there is a direct relationship between force and acceleration (i.e., F_{NET} a), then as the force applied to a body increases, the acceleration the body undergoes will also increase.

10. A negative acceleration (also known as a "deceleration") means the body is slowing down.

11. Given: KE = 10 joules

m = 5 kg

v = ?

$$KE = \frac{1}{2}\ m\ v^2 \qquad\qquad NOTE:\ 1\ J = \frac{kg\text{-}m^2}{s^2}$$

$$10J = \frac{1}{2}\ (5\ kg)\ v^2$$

$$v^2 = \frac{2\ (10J)}{5\ kg} = 4\frac{m^2}{s^2} \qquad NOTE:\ \frac{J}{kg} = \frac{\frac{kg\text{-}m^2}{s^2}}{kg} = \frac{m^2}{s^2}$$

$$v = \sqrt{4\frac{m^2}{s^2}} = 2\frac{m}{s}$$

12.
$$Given: \quad m = 9.1 \times 10^{-31} kg$$

$$c = 3 \times 10^8 \frac{m}{s}$$

$$E = mc^2$$

$$= (9.1 \times 10^{-31} \ kg)(3 \times 10^8 \ \frac{m}{s})^2$$

$$= (9.1 \times 10^{-31} \ kg)(9 \times 10^{16} \frac{m^2}{s^2})$$

$$= 8.19 \times 10^{-14} \ joules$$

$$(8.19 \times 10^{-14} \ joules) \times 1 \frac{eV}{1.6 \times 10^{-19} \ joules} \approx 5.12 \times 10^5 \ eV$$

$$= 5.12 \times 10^5 \ eV \times \frac{1 \ keV}{10^3 \ eV}$$

$$= 5.12 \ keV$$

13. Given: P = 1200 watts

t = 1 hour = 3600 seconds

E = ?

P = E/t

Solving for the energy, E:

E = P x t

   = (1200 watts)(3600 seconds)   **NOTE:** watt = joule/second

   = 4.32 x 10⁶ joules   so watt - second = joule

14. Given: E = 12,000 joules

P = 2000 watts

t = ?

Using the defining equation for power,

$$P = \frac{E}{t}$$

and solving for t:

$$t = \frac{E}{P}$$

$$= \frac{1.2 \times 10^4 \ J}{2 \times 10^3 \ watts}$$

$$= 0.6 \ x \ 10^1 \ seconds \ or \ 6 \ seconds$$

15. From the definition of power we have:

$$Power = \frac{Energy}{Time}$$

or

$$Power \times Time = Energy$$

Since the kilowatt is a unit of power and the hour is a unit of time, then when we have power x time, from the above we have energy. Thus the kilowatt-hour is used to measure the amount of energy used.

CHAPTER 3 SOLUTIONS

1. Particulate radiation refers to **particle** radiation (e.g., alpha, beta, positrons, and neutrons). Photon radiation refers to electromagnetic radiation such as the various forms of light (e.g., x-rays, gamma rays, microwaves, visible light, etc.) which carry energy but do not have mass.

2. The "wave-particle duality" of light refers to the fact that light behaves like a wave when it interacts with matter on the macroscopic (large scale) level. However, on the microscopic level, it behaves more like a "particle" or "packet" of pure energy known as a photon.

3. a. 2.5 waves

   b. 2 waves

   c. 1.25 waves

   d. 2 waves

4. a. The wave shown is a transverse wave.

17

b. amplitude = 4 units (i.e., maximum displacement)

c. $\lambda = \dfrac{90 \text{ cm}}{4.5 \text{ waves}} = 20$ cm

d. $f = \dfrac{3 \text{ waves}}{1.5 \text{ sec}} = 2$ Hz

e. $v = f\lambda$

   $= (2 \text{ Hz})(20 \text{ cm})$

   $= 40$ cm/sec

5. a. 1 mm x 1m/10^3 mm x 1 Å/10^{-10} m = $(1 \times 10^{-3} \times 10^{10})$ Å

                                                   = 10^7 Å

  b. 1 Å x 10^{-10} m/1 Å x 10^3 mm/1 m = $(1 \times 10^{-10} \times 10^3)$ mm

                                                   = 10^{-7} mm

6. a. $f = \dfrac{4.5 \text{ waves}}{9 \text{ sec}} = 0.5$ Hz

  b. $f = \dfrac{3 \text{ waves}}{3 \times 10^{-3}} = 1 \times 10^3$ Hz = 1000 Hz

  c. $f = \dfrac{2.25 \text{ waves}}{9 \times 10^{-6} \text{ sec}} = 0.25 \times 10^6$ Hz = 0.25 MHz

NOTE: All multiples and submultiples of metric units must be converted to basic units (e.g., seconds) before calculations are performed.

7. a. $v = \lambda f$

   $f = v/\lambda$

     $= \dfrac{3 \times 10^8 \text{ m/s}}{400 \times 10^{-9} \text{ m}}$

     $= \dfrac{3 \times 10^8 \text{ m/s}}{} = 0.75 \times 10^{15}$ Hz = 7.5×10^{14} Hz

     $= 4 \times 10^{-7}$ m

  b. $\lambda = v/f$
     $= \dfrac{3 \times 10^8 \text{ m/s}}{3 \times 10^{19} \text{ Hz}} = 1 \times 10^{-11}$ m or 0.1 Å

8. a. $E(\text{keV}) = \dfrac{12.4}{\lambda(\text{Å})}$

$$= \frac{12.4}{0.177 \ \text{\AA}} = 70 \text{ keV}$$

b. $E(keV) = \dfrac{12.4}{7000 \ \text{\AA}} = 1.77 \times 10^{-3}$ keV or 1.77 eV

c. $E(keV) = \dfrac{12.4}{24.8 \ \text{\AA}} = 0.5$ keV or 500 eV

d. $E(keV) = \dfrac{12.4}{0.05 \text{\AA}} = 248$ keV

e. a, c, and e are ionizing since they exceed 33-35 eV. Only b would be classified as nonionizing.

9. a. $^{12}_{6}C$ (carbon)

b. $^{182}_{74}W$ (tungsten)

c. $^{98}_{42}Mo$ (molybdenum)

d. $^{3}_{1}H$ (tritium)

10.

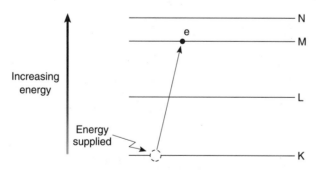

b. Binding energies are indicated as negatives to indicate that this is energy which must be **supplied** to remove an electron from the individual shells.

c. 25 keV is required for the K-shell.

20 eV is required for the N-shell.

The great difference between these two values results from the fact that electrons in the K-shell are held more tightly to the atom since they are closer to the attractive force of the nucleus.

d. $E_A = E_4 - E_3$

$= -20 \text{ eV} - (-30 \text{ eV})$

$= -20 \text{ eV} + 30 \text{ eV}$

$= 10 \text{ eV}$

Photon A is not ionizing since it is **less** than 33-35 eV.

e. $E_B = E_4 - E_1$

$= -20 \text{ eV} - (-25 \text{ keV})$

$= -0.020 \text{ keV} + 25 \text{ keV}$

$= 24.98 \text{ keV}$

Photon B is ionizing since its energy exceeds 33-35 eV.

11. Photon A is designated as a M_α x-ray.

Photon B is designated as an K_β x-ray.

Photon C is designated as a L_α x-ray.

Photon D is designated as a L_β x-ray.

12. a. 12 nucleons, 7 protons, 7 electrons, 5 neutrons, nitrogen

b. 60 nucleons, 27 protons, 27 electrons, 33 neutrons, cobalt

c. 96 nucleons, 42 protons, 42 electrons, 54 neutrons, molybdenum

d. 127 nucleons, 53 protons, 53 electrons, 74 neutrons, iodine

e. 186 nucleons, 74 protons, 74 electrons, 112 neutrons, tungsten

13. a. alphas

  b. gamma rays

  c. negatrons

  d. positrons

  e. negatrons

  f. alphas

  g. alpha, negatrons, positrons

  h. photon radiation (e.g., x-rays, gammas, IR, UV, radiowaves, visible light, etc.)

  i. characteristic x-rays

  j. gamma rays

14. $A = (5000 \text{ Ci})(0.5)^{13.25 \text{ yrs}/5.3 \text{ yrs}}$

$= (5000 \text{ Ci})(0.5)^{2.5}$

$\approx (5000 \text{ Ci})(0.18)$

$= 900 \text{ Ci}$

15. $A = A_o (0.5)^N$

$A/A_o = (0.5)^N$

$0.0625 = (0.5)^N$

$\ln(0.0625) = N \ln(0.5)$

$-2.77 = N(-0.693)$

$N = \dfrac{-2.77}{-0.693} = 4 \text{ physical half-lives}$

16. From the graph:

  a. $\sim 1.75 \ T_{1/2}\text{s}$

  b. $\sim 1.65\%$

  c. $\text{time} = (0.31 \ T_{1/2}\text{s})(20 \text{ days}/T_{1/2}) = 6.2 \text{ days}$

EXERCISE SOLUTIONS

1. a. $\lambda = \dfrac{80 \text{ nm}}{4 \text{ waves}} = 20 \text{ nm}$

   $f = \dfrac{4 \text{ waves}}{20 \times 10^{-6} \text{ sec}} = 200,000 \text{ Hz or } 200 \text{ kHz}$

   $v = (20 \text{ nm})(2 \times 10^5 \text{ Hz})$

   $= (2 \times 10^{-8}\text{m})(2 \times 10^5 \text{ Hz})$

   $= 4 \times 10^{-3} \text{ m/s or } 4 \text{ mm/s}$

   b. $\lambda = \dfrac{3 \text{ mm}}{1.5 \text{ waves}} = 2 \text{ mm}$

   $f = \dfrac{1.5 \text{ waves}}{10 \times 10^{-3} \text{ sec}} = 1.5 \times 10^2 \text{ Hz} = 150 \text{ Hz}$

   $v = (2 \text{ mm})(150 \text{ Hz}) = 300 \text{ mm/sec or } 0.3 \text{ m/s}$

   c. $\lambda = \dfrac{3\mu\text{m}}{0.5 \text{ waves}} = 6 \text{ m}$

   $f = \dfrac{0.5 \text{ waves}}{5 \times 10^{-6} \text{ sec}} = 10^5 \text{ Hz or } 100 \text{ kHz}$

   $v = (6 \times 10^{-6}\text{m})(10^5 \text{ Hz}) = 6 \times 10^{-1} \text{ m/s or } 0.6 \text{ m/s}$

2. a. $\lambda f = c$

   $f = c/\lambda$

   $= \dfrac{3 \times 10^8 \text{ m/s}}{5500 \times 10^{-10} \text{ m}}$

   $= \dfrac{3 \times 10^8 \text{ m/s}}{5.5 \times 10^{-7} \text{ m}} = 5.45 \times 10^{14} \text{ Hz}$

   $E(\text{keV}) = \dfrac{12.4}{\lambda (\text{Å})}$

   $= \dfrac{12.4}{5500 \text{ Å}}$

   $= 0.00225 \text{ keV or } 2.25 \text{ eV}$

   b. $f = c/\lambda$

   $= \dfrac{3 \times 10^8 \text{ m/s}}{10^{-2} \text{ m}}$

   $= 3 \times 10^{10} \text{ Hz}$

$$E(keV) = \frac{12.4}{\lambda(\AA)}$$

$$= \frac{12.4}{10^8 \, \AA}$$

$$= 12.4 \times 10^{-8} \text{ keV or } 1.24 \times 10^{-4} \text{ eV}$$

c. $f = c/\lambda$

$$= \frac{3 \times 10^8 \text{ m/s}}{7 \text{ m}} \approx 4.29 \times 10^7 \text{ Hz}$$

$$= E(keV) = \frac{12.4}{\lambda(\AA)}$$

$$= \frac{12.4}{7 \times 10^{10} \, \AA} = 1.77 \times 10^{-10} \text{ keV or } 1.77 \times 10^{-7} \text{ eV}$$

d. $f = c/\lambda$

$$= \frac{3 \times 10^8 \text{ m/s}}{1.77 \times 10^{-2} \times 10^{-9} \text{ m}}$$

$$= \frac{3 \times 10^8 \text{ m/s}}{1.77 \times 10^{-11} \text{ m}} \approx 1.69 \times 10^{19} \text{ Hz}$$

$$E(keV) = \frac{12.4}{\lambda(\AA)}$$

$$= \frac{12.4}{1.77 \times 10^{-1} \, \AA} \approx 70 \text{ keV}$$

3. a. 30 keV is required for the K-shell.

   500 eV is required for the M-shell.

   b. $E_A = E_4 - E_2$

   $$= -80 \text{ eV} - (-10 \text{ keV})$$

   $$= -0.08 \text{ keV} + 10 \text{ keV}$$

   $$= 9.92 \text{ keV}$$

   This would be designated as an L_β x-ray.

   c. $E_B = E_4 - E_3$

   $$= -80 \text{ eV} - (-500 \text{ eV})$$

   $$= -80 \text{ eV} + 500 \text{ eV}$$

   $$= 420 \text{ eV}$$

This would be designated as an M_α x-ray.

d. $E_c = E_4 - E_1$

$= -800\ eV - (-30\ keV)$

$= -0.08\ keV + 30\ keV$

$= 29.92\ keV$

e. Each of the x-rays shown are ionizing since their energies exceed 33-35 eV.

4. Activity remaining
as a result of decay $= A_o\ (0.5)^N$

$= (10\ mCi)(0.5)^{4\ hrs/6\ hrs}$

$= (10\ mCi)(0.5)^{0.67}$

$= (10\ mCi)(0.63)$

$= 6.3\ mCi$

Activity remaining in
patient at time of scan $= 6.3\ mCi - 4\ mCi$

$= 2.3\ mCi$

5. a. $A = A_o\ (0.5)^N$

$A/A_o = (0.5)^N$

$0.10 = (0.5)^N$

$\ln (0.10) = N \ln (0.5)$

$-2.303 = N\ (-0.693)$

$N = \dfrac{-2.303}{-0.693} = 3.3\ T_{1/2}s$

b. $A/A_o = (0.5)^N$

$0.01 = (0.5)^N$

$\ln (0.01) = N \ln (0.5)$

$-4.605 = N\ (-0.693)$

$N = \dfrac{-4.605}{-0.693} = 6.6\ T_{1/2}s$

6. $A = A_o \ (0.5)^N$

   $50 \ \text{Ci} = (200 \text{ mCi}) (0.5)^N$

   $0.050 \text{ mCi} = (200 \text{ mCi}) (0.5)^N$

   $\dfrac{0.050 \text{ mCi}}{200 \text{ mCi}} = (0.5)^N$

   $0.00025 = (0.5)^N$

   $\ln (0.00025) = N \ln (0.5)$

   $-8.29 = N \ (-0.693)$

   $N = 11.97 \ T_{1/2}\text{s}$

   Time required $= (11.97 \ T_{1/2}\text{s}) (8 \text{ days}/T_{1/2})$

   $\approx 95.8 \text{ days}$

7. $A/A_o = (0.5)^{10}$

   $\approx 0.00098 \text{ or } \sim 0.1\% \text{ remaining}$

   For a 10 Ci source, activity remaining would be:

   $A = (10 \text{ Ci}) (0.1\%)$

   $= (10 \text{ Ci}) (0.001)$

   $= 0.01 \text{ Ci or } 10 \text{ mCi}$

This rule is valid for sources having low initial activities but may not be valid for larger initial activities.

CHAPTER 4 SOLUTIONS

1. The **Coulomb** is the SI unit of electric charge.

2. # of electrons $= \dfrac{-1.6 \text{ C}}{-1.6 \times 10^{-19} \text{ C/e}}$

   $= 10^{19} \text{ electrons}$

3. The Coulomb force is **attractive** when the two charges are of **unlike** sign and repulsive when the charges are of like sign.

4. a.

$$F_c = k\frac{q_1 q_2}{d_2}$$

$$= \left(9 \times 10^9 \frac{N\text{-}m^2}{C^2}\right)\frac{(1\ C)\ (1\ C)}{(0.5\ m)^2}$$

$$= 3.6 \times 10^{10}\ Newtons \qquad\qquad (repulsive)$$

b.

$$F_c' = \left(9 \times 10^9 \frac{N\text{-}m^2}{C^2}\right)\frac{(1\ C)\ (1\ C)}{(1\ m)}$$

$$= 9 \times 10^9\ Newtons \qquad\qquad (repulsive)$$

c.

$$F_c'' = \left(9 \times 10^9 \frac{N\text{-}m^2}{C^2}\right)\frac{(1\ C)\ (1\ C)}{(1.5\ m)^2}$$

$$= 4 \times 10^9\ Newtons$$

d.

$$\frac{F_c'}{F_c} = \frac{9 \times 10^9 N}{3.6 \times 10^{10} N} = 0.25\ or\ \frac{1}{4}$$

$$\frac{F_c''}{F_c} = \frac{4 \times 10^9 N}{3.6 \times 10^{10} N} = 0.111\ or\ \frac{1}{9}$$

Thus F'$_c$ is 1/4 F$_c$ and F"$_c$ is 1/9 F$_c$. This results from the fact that F'c is **double** the separation distance of F$_c$ and F"$_c$ is **triple** the separation distance of F$_c$. The factors of 1/4 and 1/9 come from the **inverse square** relationship with distance of Coulomb's Law.

5. steel-conductor; rubber-insulator; plastic-insulator; copper-conductor; saline-conductor; glass-insulator; iron-conductor; wood-insulator; wool-insulator

6.

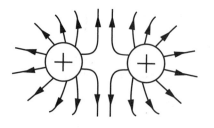

7. Electric field lines are determined by determining the direction of the electric force exerted on a small **positive** charge.

8. The total charge flowing would be:

$$q = (2 \times 10^6 \text{ electrons})(1.6 \times 10^{-19} \text{ C/e})$$

$$= 3.2 \times 10^{-13} \text{C}$$

Therefore $I = q/t$

$$= \frac{3.2 \times 10^{-13} \text{C}}{0.5 \text{ sec}}$$

$$= 6.4 \times 10^{-13} \text{ C/s}$$

$$= 6.4 \times 10^{-13} \text{ amps}$$

9. Under ordinary conditions, in order for a current to flow there must be: 1) a complete path and 2) a difference of potential between points in the path (i.e., a source of **voltage**)

10. Resistance of a wire is determined by 1) the material **composition** of the wire, 2) the **length** of the wire and 3) the thickness of the wire as measured by its cross sectional area.

11. Ohm's Law states $V = IR$. If R is constant, then $V = I$ (constant). Thus for this case as V is increased, I will correspondingly increase. That is, an increase in voltage will produce a corresponding increase in current flow.

12. a. **rheostat** is a variable resistance placed in an electric circuit to control or direct current flow.

     b. A *capacitor* is a device placed in a circuit to store electric charge until it is needed.

13. RC time constant = R x C

$$= (10^3 \text{ }\Omega)(10\mu\text{F})$$

$$= (10^3 \text{ }\Omega)(10 \times 10^{-6} \text{ F})$$

$$= 10^{-2} \text{ sec}$$

27

14. $$P = VI$$

$$100 \; watts = (120 \; volts) \; I$$

$$I = \frac{100 \; W}{120 \; V} = 0.83 \; amps$$

15. $P = I^2 R$

   $= (5A)^2 (100 \; \Omega)$

   $= 2500 \; watts$

EXERCISE SOLUTIONS

1. Current = 100 mA

   $$= 10^2 \times 10^{-3} \; \frac{coulombs}{sec}$$

   $$= 10^{-1} \; \frac{coulombs}{sec}$$

   Number of electrons/sec. $= \dfrac{10^{-1} \; C/sec}{1.6 \times 10^{-19} \; C/e-}$

   $= 6.25 \times 10^{17}$ electrons/sec

2 a.
   $$F_E = k \frac{q_1 q_2}{d^2}$$

   $$= \left(9 \times 10^9 \; \frac{N\text{-}m^2}{C^2} \right) \frac{(1.6 \times 10^{-19} \; C)^2}{(10^{-2} m)^2}$$

   $= 2.3 \times 10^{-24}$ *Newtons*   (*repulsive*)

   b. some magnitude as (a) but attractive since both electron and

   proton have the same charge magnitude

3. $F_G = G \dfrac{m_1 m_2}{d^2}$

   $$= \left(6.67 \times 10^{-11} \; \frac{N\text{-}m^2}{kg^2} \right) \frac{(1.67 \times 10^{-27} kg)(9.1 \times 10^{-31} kg)}{(10^{-2} m)^2}$$

   $= 1.01 \times 10^{-63}$ Newtons

NOTE: The gravitational force of attraction between the two particles

28

is **much** smaller than the electrical force of attraction, in fact some
2.3 x 10³⁷ times smaller due to the extremely small masses of the
electron and proton.

4. It is the electrical force of attraction between the electrons and
    the positively charged nucleus which provides the force to bind
    electrons to the atom. Due to the inverse square relationship
    with distance, this binding force decreases rapidly as electrons
    are positioned in orbits farther away from the nucleus.

5. The packet dosimeter is designed such that it reads "zero exposure"
    when the device is fully charge. If the device is used under high
    humidity conditions; charge could be neutralized and the indicator
    would begin to migrate across the scale indicating a **higher**
    exposure than that actually obtained.

6.

7. a.

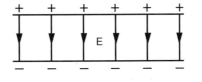

b. A proton would move from positive to negative.

c. An electron would move from negative to positive.

8. a. watt = volt x ampere

$$= \frac{joule}{coulomb} \times \frac{coulomb}{sec}$$

$$= joule/sec$$

watt = watt

b. watt = $(ampere)^2$ x ohm

$$= ampere^2 \times \frac{volt}{ampere} \qquad Recall: R = V/I$$

$$= ampere \times volt$$

$$= \frac{coulomb}{sec} \times \frac{joule}{coulomb}$$

$$= joule/sec$$

watt ≡ watt

c. joules = watts x seconds

$$= joules/sec \times seconds$$

joules ≡ joules

9. For highest resistance the wire should be **long** and **thin** (i.e., having a small cross sectional area)

10. Before any calculations are performed, the cross sectional area must first be converted to M^2 since ρ is in units of Ω-meters:

$$2\,cm^2 \times \left(\frac{1\ m}{10^2\ cm}\right)^2 = 2 \times 10^{-4} m^2$$

a. $R = \rho \frac{L}{A}$

$$R_{copper} = (1.7 \times 10^{-8}\ \Omega\text{-m})\ \frac{10m}{2\ \times\ 10^{-4} m^2}$$

$$= 8.5 \times 10^{-4}$$

b. $R_{platinum} = (1.2 \times 10^{-8} \; \Omega\text{-m}) \; \dfrac{10m}{2 \times 10^{-4}m^2}$

    $= 6 \times 10^{-4} \; \Omega$

c. $R_{glass} = (1 \times 10^{12} \Omega\text{-m}) \; \dfrac{10m}{2 \times 10^{-4}m^2}$

    $= 5 \times 10^{16}$

From the results, the best conductor (i.e., the one with the **lowest** resistance) is platinum and the worst is glass.

11.   a. $R_T = R_1 + R_2 + R_3$

      $= 2 \; \Omega + 8 \; \Omega + 10 \; \Omega$

      $= 20 \; \Omega$

    b. $V_T = I_T R_T$

      $I_T = \dfrac{V_T}{R_T}$

      $= \dfrac{20 \text{ volts}}{20 \; \Omega} = 1 \text{ amp}$

    c. $I_1 = I_2 = I_3 = I_T = 1 \text{ amp}$

      (the same current flow through each resistance)

    d. Using Ohm's Law, we have:

      $V_1 = I_1 R_1$

        $= (1 \text{ A})(2 \; \Omega)$

        $= 2 \text{ volts}$

      $V_2 = I_2 R_2$

        $= (1A)(8 \; \Omega)$

        $= 8 \text{ volts}$

      $V_3 = I_3 R_3$

        $= (1A)(10 \; \Omega)$

        $= 10 \text{ volts}$

NOTE: As a check, V_T should equal $V_1 + V_2 + V_3$ and here it does.

12. a. $1/R_T = 1/R_1 + 1/R_2$

$\qquad = 1/6 \ \Omega + 1/12 \ \Omega$

$\qquad = 2/12 \ \Omega + 1/12 \ \Omega$

$\qquad = 3/12 \ \Omega$

$\quad R_T = 12 \ \Omega/3$ or $4 \ \Omega$

b. $V_T = I_T R_T$

$\quad I_T = \dfrac{V_T}{R_T}$

$\qquad = \dfrac{12 \text{ volts}}{4 \ \Omega}$

$\qquad = 3$ amps

c. $V_1 = V_2 = V_T = 12$ volts

(since voltage is constant in parallel circuits)

d. From Ohm's Law:

$V = IR$

$I = V/R$

$I_1 = V/R_1$

$\qquad = \dfrac{12 \text{ volts}}{6 \ \Omega}$

$\qquad = 2$ amps

$I_2 = \dfrac{V}{R_2}$

$\qquad \dfrac{12 \text{ volts}}{12 \ \Omega}$

$\qquad = 1$ amp

NOTE: As a check, I_T should equal $I_1 + I_2$, and here it does. Also, note that the larger current flows through the branch (R_1) having the smaller resistance.

13. a. Recalling that **one complete AC cycle** is as shown below:

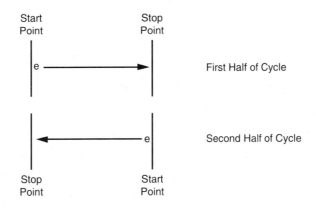

Thus the electron starts and stops **twice** during each cycle. Therefore
it starts and stops 2(60) or 120 times for 60 cycle AC and 2(50) or 100
times for 50 cycle AC.

14. Power = $\dfrac{Energy}{Time}$

   P = E/t

   t = E/P

   = $\dfrac{6 \times 10^5 joules}{1250\ watts}$

   = 480 seconds or 8 minutes

15. seconds $\stackrel{?}{=}$ Ohms x farads

   $\stackrel{?}{=}$ $\dfrac{volts}{amps}$ x $\dfrac{coulombs}{volt}$

   $\stackrel{?}{=}$ $\dfrac{coulombs}{amps}$

   $\stackrel{?}{=}$ coulombs x $\dfrac{second}{coulombs}$

   seconds ≡ seconds

33

CHAPTER 5 SOLUTIONS

1. Electric and magnetic forces are both:

    a. attractive or repulsive

    b. dependent upon the magnitude (i.e., size or strength) of the electric charges or magnetic poles

    c. inversely related to the *square* of the distance which separates the electric charges or magnetic poles

2. "Ferromagnetic" refers to materials which can be easily magnetized. Ferromagnetic materials include iron, nickel and cobalt.

3. Magnetic north and south poles cannot be separated because their origin lies in *moving electric charge*. Even an atom which has net magnetic properties as a result of its moving electrons, protons, and neutrons will have both a north and a south magnetic pole.

4. Magnetic field line direction at any point in space is defined to be the direction of the magnetic force exerted on a small hypothetical unit *NORTH* pole.

5. Magnetic field lines travel from *north* to *south outside* a bar magnet but from *south* to *north inside* the bar magnet.

6.
    a. Electric field only.

    b. An electric and a magnetic field (since the charge is moving)

    c. Magnetic field only.

    d. Magnetic field only.

    e. Neither (since the bar is neither charged nor magnetized)

    f. An electric and a magnetic field

7.

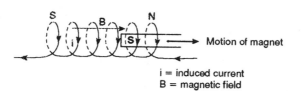

i = induced current
B = magnetic field

Explanation: As th e south pole is withdrawn from the coil, by
Lenz's Law the polarity of the coil must *oppose* the change in the
magnetic field which induces the current in the coil. To *oppose*
the withdrawal of the south pole, the right end of the coil must
act as a *north* pole (in an attempt to keep the south pole in the
coil). The left end of the coil will then become a *south* pole.
Since the coil now acts as a bar magnet, magnetic field lines
inside the coil travel from *south to north* (as shown above). Now
using the right hand rule, with the curled fingers of the right
hand placed inside the coil in the direction of the magnetic field
(**B**) lines, the thumb points downward. Thus the current (i)
induced in the coil will flow down the outside of the coil as
indicated.

8   a. No magnetic field (stationary electric charges have electric
         fields only)

     b.

     c.

     d.

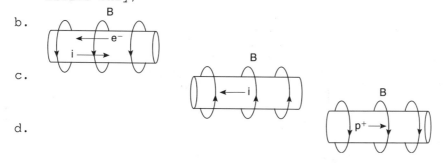

9   a. When an electric charge is put into *motion*, a magnetic field
         is produced.

     b. When a *changing* magnetic field is passed over a conductor, a
         current will be produced in the conductor.

35

c. Electric currents (AC) are used to generate magnetic fields which are in turn used to rotate components of electric motors (e.g., induction motors, synchronous motors for timers, etc.) Changing magnetic fields are used to induce currents in electrical generators and transformers.

10 a.

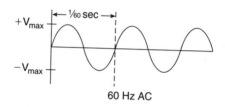

b.

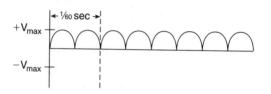

c.

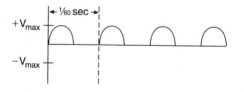

11 a.

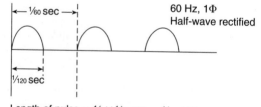

60 Hz, 1Φ
Half-wave rectified

Length of pulse = ½ × 1/60 sec = 1/120 sec

36

b.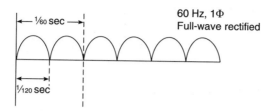

60 Hz, 1Φ
Full-wave rectified

1/60 sec

1/120 sec

Length of pulse = ½ × 1/60 sec = 1/120 sec

c.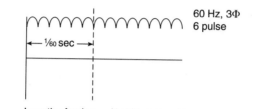

60 Hz, 3Φ
6 pulse

1/60 sec

Length of pulse = ⅙ × 1/60 sec = 1/360 sec

12. 3φ generators provide a near constant voltage. 1φ generators provide voltage which fluctuates from some peak value (V_p) to zero. 3φ generators are the attempt to obtain a *constant* voltage, which is greatly desired in the production of diagnostic x-rays of near constant energy.

13 a. 100% ripple (since the voltage drops periodically to zero)

    b. 13.5% ripple

    c. 3.5% ripple

    d. 100% ripple

14. Minimum Voltage = 120 kV - 0.10 (120 kV)

                     = 120 kV - 12 kV

                     = 108 kV

15. A low ripple factor implies that the voltage drop is also low. Thus the generator with the lowest ripple factor will provide the more constant voltage.

16   a.   step-up (turns ratio greater than one)

       b.   step-up (more turns on the secondary than on the primary)

       c.   step-down (more turns on the primary than the secondary)

       d.   step-down (turns ratio less than one)

17   a.

$$Given: \quad \frac{N_s}{N_p} = 5000$$

$$V_p = 10 \ volts$$

$$V_s = ?$$

$$\frac{V_s}{V_p} = \frac{N_s}{N_p}$$

$$\frac{V_s}{10 \ volts} = 5000$$

$$V_s = (5000)(10 \ volts) = 50 \ kV$$

       b.

$$\frac{I_p}{I_s} = \frac{N_s}{N_p}$$

$$\frac{25 \ A}{I_s} = 5000$$

$$I_s = \frac{25 \ A}{5000} = 5 \times 10^{-3} \ A \ or \ 5 \ mA$$

18   a.

$$Power \ Rating_{3\phi} = \frac{kV \times mA}{1000}$$

$$= \frac{(100 \ kV)(600 \ mA)}{1000}$$

$$= 60 \ kW$$

       b.

$$Power \ Rating_{1\phi} = \frac{0.7 \ kV \times mA}{1000}$$

$$= \frac{(0.7)(100 \ kV)(600 \ mA)}{1000}$$

$$= 42 \ kW$$

19   a. $V_{RMS} = 0.707 \ V_p$

$$= 0.707 \ (100 \ kV)$$

$$= 70.7 \ kV$$

b. $V_{RMS} = 0.707\,(70\ kV)$

$\approx 49.5\ kV$

EXERCISE SOLUTIONS

1 a. The needle will be deflected since moving charged particles produce a magnetic field.

   b. same as "a".

   c. The needle will not be deflected since a stationary charge will produce only an electric field.

   d. same as "c".

2. A simple electromagnet consists of a current carrying coil of wire which is normally wrapped around a ferromagnetic (e.g., iron) core. The electromagnet acquires its magnetic properties only when a current flows through the coils. The strength of this type of magnet is dependent upon the number of coils of wire used and the magnitude of the current which flows through them. A permanent magnet is simply a mass of some material which has been magnetized. The strength of this type magnet is dependent upon the degree of alignment of its magnetic domains. Its magnetic properties cannot be turned off.

3. Wrapping the coils of wire of an electromagnet around a ferromagnetic can enhance or strengthen the magnetic properties of the electromagnet by additionally magnetizing the core during use.

4 a.

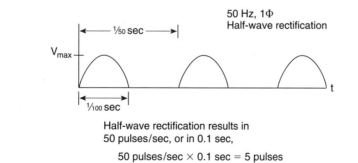

Half-wave rectification results in
50 pulses/sec, or in 0.1 sec,

50 pulses/sec $\times$ 0.1 sec = 5 pulses

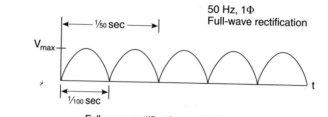

50 Hz, 1Φ
Full-wave rectification

b.

V_{max}

1/50 sec

1/100 sec

Full-wave rectification results in
100 pulses/sec, or in 0.1 sec,

100 pulses/sec × 0.1 sec = 10 pulses

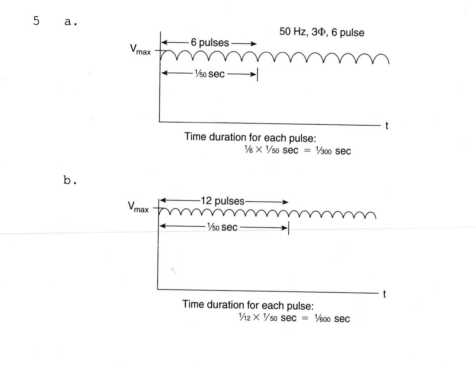

5   a.

V_{max}

6 pulses   50 Hz, 3Φ, 6 pulse

1/50 sec

t

Time duration for each pulse:
1/6 × 1/50 sec = 1/300 sec

b.

V_{max}

12 pulses

1/50 sec

t

Time duration for each pulse:
1/12 × 1/50 sec = 1/600 sec

6   a. Minimum Voltage₆ = 150 kV - .135(150 kV)

= 150 kV - 20.25 kV

= 129.75 kV

b. Minimum Voltage$_{12}$ = 150 kV - 0.035 (150 kV)

$\qquad\qquad\qquad$ = 150 kV - 5.25 kV

$\qquad\qquad\qquad$ = 144.75 kV

7. All 1ϕ generators produce voltages which fluctuate from some peak voltage (V_p) to zero. Since the voltage drops from V_p to 0, this corresponds to a 100% ripple factor.

8. High frequency generators provide an even more approximately constant voltage which is most desirous in supplying voltage to the x-ray tube. A constant, non-fluctuating voltage results in more higher energy x-rays being produced.

9. For proper operation of a transformer, there must be changing magnetic fields that originate in the primary and cut across the coils of the secondary. Once a DC current is established in the primary, its associated magnetic field becomes stabilized and does not change. If an AC current is used, its associated magnetic field changes continuously as the current continuously changes its direction. This assures proper operation of the transformer.

10   a. $\dfrac{N_s}{N_p} = \dfrac{I_p}{I_s}$

$\qquad$ $\dfrac{500}{50} = \dfrac{2\ amps}{I_s}$

$\qquad\qquad$ $I_s = \dfrac{2\ amps}{10} = 0.2\ amps$

     b. $\qquad$ $\dfrac{V_s}{V_p} = \dfrac{N_s}{N_p}$

$\qquad$ $\dfrac{10\ volts}{V_p} = 0.002$

$\qquad\qquad$ $V_p = \dfrac{10\ volts}{0.002} = 5000\ volts$

c.
$$\frac{I_s}{I_p} = \frac{V_s}{V_p}$$

$$\frac{10\ amps}{I_p} = \frac{100\ kV}{0.220\ kV}$$

$$I_p = \frac{0.220\ kV}{100\ kV} \times 10\ amps$$

$$= 0.022\ amps\ or\ 22\ mA$$

d.
$$\frac{I_p}{I_s} = \frac{N_s}{N_p}$$

$$\frac{15\ amps}{0.1\ amps} = \frac{N_s}{N_p}$$

$$\frac{N_s}{N_p} = turns\ ratio = 150$$

Note: In both "c" and "d" multiples of basic units must be converted to the same units *prior* to performing calculations.

11.
$$Power\ rating_{3\phi} = \frac{kV \times mA}{1000}$$

$$30\ kW = \frac{(70\ kV)\ (current\ in\ mA)}{1000}$$

$$current\ (mA) = \frac{(30\ kW)\ (1000)}{(70\ kV)}$$

$$= 428.6\ mA$$

CHAPTER 6 SOLUTIONS

1. Adequate vacuum conditions within the x-ray tube are required to maintain a clear path for the extremely light electrons as they travel from the filament to the target. Collisions between these electrons and any air molecules would decrease the number of electrons striking the target and the number of resulting x-rays produced.

2. a. The glass envelope provides mechanical support for the x-ray tube components and maintains the vacuum conditions

necessary for proper tube operation.

b. The cathode is the negative electrode of the x-ray tube. This electrode along with the anode is necessary to provide the kilovoltage required for x-ray production.

c. The filament is the source of electrons within the x-ray tube. These electrons are required for x-ray production.

d. An appropriate target with which fast moving electrons will collide is required for x-ray production.

e. The anode is the positive electrode of the x-ray. This electrode along with the cathode is necessary to provide the kilovoltage required to accelerate electrons into the target to produce x-rays.

f. The focusing cup is required to prevent the divergence or spreading of the stream of electrons as they are emitted from the filament and move toward the anode target.

3. Rotating anode tubes have the capability of safely handling radiographic procedures which generate greater quantities of heat (e.g., higher mA procedures, rapid multiple exposures, etc.) than do tubes with stationary anodes which cannot dissipate heat as rapidly.

4. As the kilovoltage is increased, the electrons move faster toward the anode target. The faster the electrons are moving as they strike the target, the more penetrating the x-rays produced.

5. Fans force air to circulate and as a result heat is removed via forced convection. Both circulating air and circulating oil are used to transfer heat from an x-ray tube using the method of heat transfer known as convection.

6. The line focus principle makes use of a target which is slanted at an angle to the vertical. By slanting the target, the heat generated at the target plate is distributed over a larger area which assists in heat dissipation. The tilt of the target plate also reduces the focal spot size from which x-rays appear to originate. This smaller "effective focal spot" results in sharper image production.

7. a. HU = (1.35)(kVp)(mA)(sec)

    = (1.35)(70 kVp)(200 mA)(0.5 sec)

    = 9450 HU

    b. HU = (1.41)(kVp)(mA)(sec)

    = (1.41)(80 kVp)((100 mA)(0.1 sec)

    = 1128 HU

    c. HU = (1.41)(kVp)(mA)(sec)

    = (1.41)(100 kVp)(800 mA)(0.5 sec)

    = 56,400 HU

    d. HU = (kVp)(mA)(sec)

    = (100 kVp)(300 mA)(1 sec)

    = 30,000 HU

    e. HU = (1.35)(kVp)(mA)(sec)

    = (1.35)(60 kVp)(1000 mA)(0.8 sec)

    = 64,800 HU

8. a. Unacceptable

    b. Acceptable

    c. Unacceptable

    d. Acceptable

    e. Unacceptable

f. Unacceptable

g. Acceptable

9. From the anode cooling curve shown, it takes 14 minutes for the anode to cool when the maximum 240,000 HU have been deposited. When lower quantities of heat are deposited, it will cool in the times indicated below:

a. Time to cool = 14 min - 1.2 min

        = 12.8 min

Note: This is determined by locating the number of heat units deposited on the vertical axis. Move horizontally from this point to the cooling curve. Drop a vertical line to the horizontal (time) axis from this point. Subtract this time from the 14 minute maximum cooling time.

b. Time to cool = 14 min - 5.2 min

        = 8.8 min

c. Time to cool = 14 min - 10.8 min

        = 3.2 min

EXERCISE SOLUTIONS

1. Assuming all other physical factors remain unchanged,

a. the larger the mass of the block, the more heat the anode can handle since its temperature rise will be less (recall $\Delta T = Q/mc$ where ΔT = temperature change of the block, Q = heat energy added, m = mass of block, and c = specific heat)

b. the greater the diameter of a rotating anode disk, the

greater the area covered by the target track

c. the higher the rotational speed of the anode, the shorter the time that any one point on the target is bombarded by the incident beam of electrons which is the source of heat generation

2. Recalling that the resistance of a conducting wire is directly related to its length and inversely related to its cross-sectional area (i.e., $R = \rho L/A$), electrical resistance can be maximized by using a long, thin wire. High electrical resistance will produce heat in the filament which is needed for electron production by thermionic emission.

3. a. From the input curve, a procedure which delivers 350 HU/sec can be conduced for 14 minutes without exceeding the maximum anode heat storage capacity of 240,000 HU since the input curve does not approach this upper limit after 14 min.

    Answer: Yes

    From the 350 HU/sec input curve, after 14 minutes the anode would have stored approximately **140,000 HU.**

    Now using the cooling curve, the time to cool after the deposition of 140,000 HU would be 14 min - 2.2 min = **11.8 min**

b. Using the 500 HU/sec input curve, approximately **180,000 HU** will be deposited in the anode after 9 min.

Using the cooling curve, it will take

14 min - 1.2 min = **12.8 minutes** to cool completely.

c. Using the 250 HU/sec input curve, it will take

approximately **7.5 min** to deposit 80,000 HU.

d. Using the cooling curve, after a deposition of

180,000 HU, one minute later (from time = 1.2 min to time

= 2.2 min) the heat remaining in the anode drops to

approximately 140,000 HU. This is a cooling rate of

$$\frac{180,000 \; HU - 140,000 \; HU}{1 \; min} = 40,000 \; \frac{HU}{min}$$

When the anode holds 20,000 HU, one minute later (from

time = 10.8 min to time = 11.8 min) the heat in the

anode drops to approximately 14,000 HU. This is a

cooling rate of $$\frac{20,000 \; HU - 14,000 \; HU}{1 \; min} = 6000 \frac{HU}{min}$$

The much higher cooling rate occurs when higher

quantities of heat are stored in the anode. When the

anode is at higher temperatures, rapid heat loss occurs

via the heat transfer process of radiation. This method

of heat loss decreases rapidly as the temperature of the

anode drops.

CHAPTER 7 SOLUTIONS

1. a. The autotransformer allows the radiographer to make small

changes in the incoming line voltage which will allow the

radiographer to control the voltage (kVp) across the x-ray tube electrodes. The autotransformer also provides voltage to the x-ray filament circuit necessary to generate current flow through the filament for thermionic emission.

b. The step-up (or high voltage) transformer allows incoming line voltage which is of the order of a hundred volts or so to be stepped up to the necessary kilovoltage level required for the production of diagnostic energy x-rays.

c. The step-down transformer, located in the filament circuit, allows incoming line voltage to be stepped down from hundreds of volts to approximately 10 volts which is the level necessary to generate sufficient current in the filament for thermionic emission.

d. Rectifiers are needed to convert AC voltage from the high voltage transformer to DC voltage which will be placed across the x-ray tube electrode. DC voltage is required to maintain single direction current flow between the tube electrodes to make the most efficient use of the voltage waveform in the production of x-rays.

e. Variable resistances are used in the filament circuit to allow the radiographer to vary the voltage on the primary side of the step-down transformer. This allows the radiographer to control the voltage placed across the filament and hence the filament current.

f. Voltmeters are placed in the x-ray circuit to measure the kVp across the x-ray tube electrodes.

g. Ammeters are used in the x-ray circuit to measure current flow such as the tube current (i.e., mA)

2. Line voltage refers to the voltage supplied by the local power company or power generating station to your facility.

3. The filament, being a long, thin wire, has a relatively large amount of electrical resistance (recall the resistance relationship $R = \rho$ L/A where L = length of the wire and A = the cross-sectional area of the wire). As more current is passed through the wire more heat is generated through electrical resistance. The more heat energy produced the more electrons released from the metal surface.

4. Incoming line voltage can be varied slightly (e.g., halved or doubled and points in between) by varying the turns ratio (kVp selector) of the autotransformer. This voltage which comes off the secondary of the autotransformer is then supplied to the primary of the high voltage transformer which has a fixed turns ratio. The voltage supplied by the autotransformer is then stepped up to the required kilovoltage levels. Thus by varying slightly the incoming line voltage, one can effectively vary the voltage across the x-ray tube electrodes.

5. Because of the manner in which x-ray tube voltage is varied it is very important to have a stable line voltage. Any rise or fall in incoming line voltage can result in major changes in tube voltage which will directly affect both the energy and the number of x-rays produced.

6. The autotransformer has a *variable* turns ratio which can be varied by the radiographer. Other transformers (step-up and

step-down) found in the x-ray circuit have a *fixed* turns
ratio which cannot be changed.

7. The step-up transformer, being the high voltage transformer,
    has a need for electrical insulation which is provided by
    the oil. The step-down transformer is connected to the
    filament, a part of the cathode assembly of the x-ray tube,
    which is also maintained at a high voltage. The oil acts
    again to provide electrical insulation. In addition to
    electrical insulation the oil acts as a convection fluid to
    aid in the removal of heat generated as current flows
    through the primary and secondary coils of the individual
    transformers.

8. Transformers require a *changing* current (or voltage) to
    function. Therefore transformers can function properly
    using *AC* current since the current changes its direction of
    motion and voltage reverses its polarity twice during each
    AC cycle. Batteries, however, provide only *DC* current, which
    does not change its direction of flow. Voltage supplied
    by batteries also remains constant during use.

9. For an x-ray timing device to operate properly it must
    terminate (i.e., end) the radiographic exposure after the
    passage of a specified period of time. If the exposure was
    to be terminated by turning off the filament current,
    electrons could still be emitted from the heated filament
    wire. With voltage still in place across the tube
    electrodes, these electrons could still be pulled into the
    anode and x-rays produced. Therefore the most efficient way
    to end the exposure is to remove the high voltage across the

tube electrodes. In this way no electrons will be pulled into the anode and no x-rays will be produced. Removal of the high voltage can also be accomplished almost instantaneously.

10. a. Filament current refers to the current which flows through the tube filament in order to generate sufficient heat for thermionic emission. Filament current is measured in amperes.

   b. Tube current refers to the current produced by the flow of electrons between the x-ray tube electrodes during the making of a radiographic exposure. Tube current is measured in *milliamperes* (i.e., mA).

   c. mAs is the product of tube current (mA) and exposure time (sec). Physically mAs represents current x time = (charge/time) x time = charge. Thus mAs represents the total amount of *charge* that flows between the tube electrodes during an exposure. This in turn relates to the number of electrons that move between the tube electrodes during an exposure.

11. a.

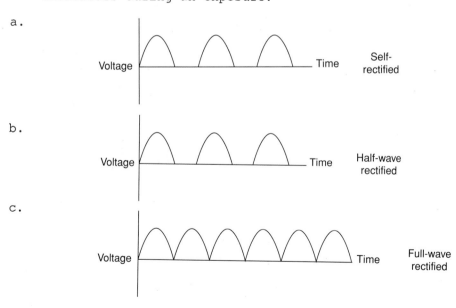

12. a. Single phase generators produce voltage waveforms which begin at 0, rise to some maximum voltage, then return to 0. This always results in a 100% ripple factor.

   b. Three phase generators produce voltage waveforms which begin at some minimum, nonzero voltage, rise to some maximum voltage, then drop back to the initial minimum, nonzero voltage. This typically results in ripple factors less than 15%.

   c. The voltage waveforms obtained with high frequency generators are similar to these obtained with three phase units but with ripple factors of approximately 4% or less.

13. Since the voltage produced by single phase rectified units always ranges from zero to some maximum voltage, the corresponding energies of the x-rays produced will also range from zero to some maximum energy. With three phase and high frequency generators the voltage drop is minimized resulting in a higher *average* energy of the x-rays produced.

14. a. 1/20 sec = 0.05 sec; this will result in a correct exposure

   b. 1/5 sec = 2/10 sec; since the unit terminated the exposure in less than the designated time, the radiograph will be underexposed

   c. 1/4 sec = 0.25 sec = 250 msec; this will result in a correct exposure

d. 1/2 sec = 0.5 sec; since the unit terminated the exposure
    after a time *longer* than the designated time, the
    radiograph will be overexposed

15. a. This will result in two (2) voltage pulses each 1/60 sec
        or 120 pulses each second

    b. This will result in one (1) voltage pulse each 1/60 sec
        or 60 pulses each second

    c. This will result in 6 pulses each 1/60 sec or 360 pulses
        each second

    d. This will result in 12 pulses each 1/60 sec or 720 pulses
        each second

16. Tube current is measured in milliamperes (mA) whereas
    filament current is measured in *amperes*.

17. Since high frequency generators use voltage having higher
    frequencies than standard 60 Hz AC, this allows for the use
    of transformers having fewer coils of wire needed to produce
    the kV levels required for diagnostic x-ray production.
    This allows for smaller, more compact x-ray units. Ripple factors
    of these units are comparable if not smaller than those of three-
    phase units. This results in higher average energy x-ray
    production.

18. Three types of generator systems used in portable x-ray units are
    battery powered units, capacitor discharge units and high
    frequency units.

19. The falling load generator is designed to use the highest mA at a
    specific kVp setting for time intervals that do not exceed the
    heat loading capabilities of the tube while still obtaining the
    desired mAs.

EXERCISE SOLUTIONS

1. a. output voltage of autotransformer would be:

$$\frac{V_s}{V_p} = \frac{N_s}{N_p}$$

$$V_s = \left(\frac{N_s}{N_p}\right) V_p$$

$$= (0.97)(120 \ volts)$$

$$= 116.4 \ volts$$

output voltage of step-up transformer and voltage supplied to the x-ray tube would be:

$$\frac{V_s}{V_p} = \frac{N_s}{N_p}$$

$$V_s = \left(\frac{N_s}{N_p}\right) V_p$$

$$= (600)(116.4 \ volts)$$

$$= 69840 \ volts \ (or \ 69.84 \ kV)$$

b. output voltage of autotransformer would be:

$$V_s = \left(\frac{N_s}{N_p}\right) V_p$$

$$= (1.25)(120 \ volts)$$

$$= 150 \ volts$$

output voltage of step-up transformer and voltage supplied to the x-ray tube would be:

c.   output voltage of autotransformer would be:

$$V_s = \left(\frac{N_s}{N_p}\right) V_p$$

$$= (1.389)(120 \; volts)$$

$$= 166.68 \; volts$$

output voltage of step-up transformer and voltage supplied to the x-ray tube would be:

$$V_s = \left(\frac{N_s}{N_p}\right) V_p$$

$$= (600)(166.68 \; volts)$$

$$= 100,008 \; volts \; (or \approx 100 \; kV)$$

2.

$$Ripple \; factor = \frac{V_{MAX} - V_{MIN}}{V_{MAX}} \times 100\%$$

a. $Ripple \; factor = \dfrac{90 \; kV - 78.3 \; kV}{90 \; kV} \times 100\% = 13\%$

b. $Ripple \; factor = \dfrac{100 \; kV - 0}{100\%} \times 100\% = 100\%$

c. $Ripple \; factor = \dfrac{80 \; kV - 77.6 \; kV}{80 \; kV} \times 100\% = 3\%$

3.

a. $\dfrac{V_s}{V_p} = \dfrac{N_s}{N_p}$

$V_p = \left(\dfrac{N_p}{N_s}\right)(V_s)$

$= \left(\dfrac{100}{5000}\right)(80\ kV)$

$= 1.6\ kV\ or\ 1600\ volts$

b. $\dfrac{V_s}{V_p} = \dfrac{N_s}{N_p}$

$V_s = \left(\dfrac{N_s}{N_p}\right)V_p$

$= (500)(220\ volts)$

$= 110,000\ volts\ (or\ 110\ kv)$

c. $\dfrac{V_s}{V_p} = \dfrac{N_s}{N_p} = Turns\ ratio$

$Turns\ ratio = \dfrac{V_s}{V_p}$

$= \dfrac{66,000\ volts}{120\ volts}$

$= 550$

d. $\dfrac{V_s}{V_p} = \dfrac{N_s}{N_p}$

$\quad V_s = \left(\dfrac{N_s}{N_p}\right)V_p$

$\quad\quad = \left(\dfrac{80,000}{200}\right)(150 \; volts)$

$\quad\quad = (400)(150 \; volts)$

$\quad\quad = 60,000 \; volts \; (or \; 60 \; kV)$

e. $\dfrac{V_s}{V_p} = \dfrac{N_s}{N_p}$

$\quad N_s = \left(\dfrac{V_s}{V_p}\right)(N_p)$

$\quad\quad = \left(95,000 \; \dfrac{volts}{190} \; volts\right)(125 \; turns)$

$\quad\quad = 62,500 \; turns$

4. Recall 1 ampere $= \; 1 \; \dfrac{coulomb}{sec}$

so,

$\quad$ 1 mA $= \; 0.001 \; \dfrac{coulomb}{sec}$

Then the number of electrons required to produce a charge of 0.001 coulomb would be:

$$\dfrac{0.001 \; coulomb}{1.6 \times 10^{-19} \; \dfrac{coulomb}{electron}} = 6.25 \times 10^{15} \; electrons$$

Therefore, since 1 mA $= \; 6.25 \times 10^{15} \; \dfrac{electrons}{sec}$, then

$\quad$ 100 $mA = 100 \times 6.25 \times 10^{15} \; \dfrac{electrons}{sec} = 6.25 \times 10^{17} \; \dfrac{electrons}{sec}$

$\quad$ 300 $mA = 300 \times 6.25 \times 10^{15} \; \dfrac{electrons}{sec} = 1.875 \times 10^{18} \; \dfrac{electrons}{sec}$

$\quad$ 1000 $mA = 1000 \times 6.25 \times 10^{15} \; \dfrac{electrons}{sec} = 6.25 \times 10^{18} \; \dfrac{electrons}{sec}$

5. a. 1φ, half-wave rectified units produce 60 x-ray pulses each second. Therefore one should observe 1/10 (60) or 6 dots on the film if the timer was accurate. Since 8 dots are observed, this indicates that the unit has been on longer than it should be (actually 8/60 sec or 0.13 sec when the timer is set for 0.1 sec). Therefore the timer is slow and will result in an overexposure.

   b. 1φ, full-wave rectified units produce 120 x-ray pulses each second. Therefore one should observe 1/5 (120) or 24 dots on the film if the timer was accurate. Since only 10 dots are observed, this indicates that the unit has been on for a shorter period of time than it should be (actually 10/120 sec or 0.08 sec rather than 0.2 sec). Therefore the timer is fast and will result in an underexposure.

   c. 1φ, full-wave rectified units produce 120 pulses each second. 1/20 sec corresponds to 0.05 sec 6 dots represent 6/120 sec or 0.05 sec. Therefore the timer should be considered accurate.

   d. 1φ, half-wave rectified units produce 60 pulses each second. 35 dots corresponds to 35/60 sec or 0.58 sec. Therefore the unit has been on longer than it should be and the timer is slow. This can result in an overexposure.

CHAPTER 8 SOLUTIONS

1. Unlike alpha and beta particles, which are charged particles and interact electrically with matter, photons are uncharged and cannot interact electrically. For this reason photons must interact with matter in a different manner.

58

2. Photons interact with matter by way of classical scattering, photoelectric, Compton scattering, pair production, triplet production or photodisintegration interactions.

3. Photoelectric, Compton scattering and triplet production all result in ionization events.

4. Diagnostic energy x-rays may interact in tissue by way of classical scattering, photoelectric or Compton scattering events.

5. Incident photons are completely absorbed in photoelectric, pair production, triplet production and photodisintegration interactions.

6. High energy photon interactions include pair production, triplet production, and photodisintegration interactions.

7. Since the photon is of *lower* energy, the scattered photon will be of *longer* wavelength and *lower* frequency than the incident photon.

8. Energy of the scatter radiation is determined by the energy of the incident photon and the angle through which the photons are scattered.

9 a. Maximum energy is transferred to the recoil electron when the photon is scattered through 180° (i.e., backscatter)

   b. The minimum energy scattered photons also occur at 180° scattering angles as a result of being maximum energy transferred to the recoil electrons.

10. Scatter radiation is always of lower energy and this increases its chances of being absorbed photoelectrically in the bodies of attending personnel. Such absorption will increase radiation dose to personnel unless appropriate radiation precautions are taken.

11. a. Only triplet production results in an ionization event for high energy photon interactions.

    b. Pair production events require the incident photon energy to be at least 1.022 MeV.

    c. Photodisintegration

    c. Triplet production requires the incident photon energy be at least 2.04 MeV.

12. For diagnostic energy x-rays, HVL ranges are

    soft tissue: 4-8 cm

    aluminum: 3-5 mm

13. The numerical value of the HVL is influenced by the energy of the incident photons and the material of which the absorber is made.

14. a. 75% of the incident beam is attenuated by 2 HVLs.

    b. 25% of the incident beam is transmitted by 2 HVLs.

15. a. Compton scattering

    b. photoelectric interactions (due to high Z number)

    c. photoelectric interactions (due to high Z number)

EXERCISE SOLUTIONS

1. A 50 keV photon cannot eject a K-shell electron since it does not have sufficient energy to overcome the K-shell electronic binding energy.

2. For photoelectric interactions:

$$E_i = E_b + E_e$$
$$90 \ keV = 88 \ keV + E_e$$
$$E_e = 90 \ keV - 88 \ keV = 2 \ keV$$

3. For Compton scattering events:

$$E_i = E_b + E_e + E_s$$

$$70 \ keV = 0 + 25 \ keV + E_s$$

$$E_s = 70 \ keV - 25 \ keV = 45 \ keV$$

4. Given: $E_i = 85 \ keV$

$$E_b = 800 \ eV = 0.8 \ keV$$

$$\theta = 90°$$

First use the technique shown in Special Insert 8-2 to find the energy of the scattered photon:

The wavelength of the incident photon is:

$$\lambda (\text{Å}) = \frac{12.4}{85 \ keV} \approx 0.1459 \text{Å}$$

The increase in λ of the scattered photon is:

$$\Delta (\text{Å}) = 0.024 (1 - \cos 90°)$$

$$= 0.024 (1 - 0) = 0.024 \text{Å}$$

The wavelength of the scattered photon, λ', is

$$\lambda' = \lambda + \Delta\lambda$$

$$= 0.1459 \text{Å} + 0.024 \text{Å}$$

$$\approx 0.1699 \ \text{Å}$$

Then the energy of the scattered photon is then given by:

$$E' = \frac{12.4}{0.1699 \text{Å}} \approx 73 \ keV \quad \text{← } Energy \ of \ scattered \ photon$$

Now using the general energy equation for Compton scattering events:

$$E_i = E_b + E_e + E_s$$

$$85\ keV = 0.8\ keV + E_e + 73\ keV$$

$$E_e = 85\ keV - 0.8\ keV - 73\ keV$$

$$E_e = 11.2\ keV$$

5a.

$$\lambda = \frac{12.4}{60\ keV} \approx 0.2067\text{Å}$$

$$\Delta\lambda = 0.024(1-\cos 25°)$$

$$= 0.024(1- .9063) = .024(0.0937) = 0.0022\text{Å}$$

$$\lambda' = \lambda = \Delta\lambda$$

$$= 0.2067\text{Å} + 0.0022\text{Å} = 0.2089\text{Å}$$

$$E' = \frac{12.4}{0.2089\text{Å}} \approx \textbf{59.4 keV}$$

b.

$$\lambda = \frac{12.4}{90\ keV} \approx 0.1378\text{Å}$$

$$\Delta\lambda = 0.024(1-\cos 25°) = 0.0022\text{Å}$$

$$\lambda' = 0.1378\text{Å} + 0.0022\text{Å} = 0.14\text{Å}$$

$$E' = \frac{12.4}{0.14\text{Å}} \approx \textbf{88.6 keV}$$

c.

$$\lambda = \frac{12.4}{120\ keV} \approx 0.1033\text{Å}$$

$$\Delta\lambda = 0.024(1-\cos 25°) = 0.0022\text{Å}$$

$$\lambda' = \lambda + \Delta\lambda$$

$$= 0.1033\text{Å} + 0.0022\text{Å} = 0.1055\text{Å}$$

$$E' = \frac{12.4}{0.1055\text{Å}} \approx \textbf{117.5 keV}$$

d.

$$\lambda = \frac{12.4}{160\ keV} \approx 0.0775\text{Å}$$

$$\Delta\lambda = 0.024(1-\cos 25°) = 0.0022\text{Å}$$

$$\lambda' = \lambda + \Delta\lambda$$

$$= 0.0775\text{Å} + 0.0022\text{Å} = 0.0797\text{Å}$$

$$E' = \frac{12.4}{0.0797\text{Å}} \approx \textbf{155.6 keV}$$

As the incident photon energy increases, the energy of the scatter radiation at any particlular angle also increases. Thus as the incident photon energy increases, more energetic scatter will have a greater chance of reaching the image receptor and cause a degradation of the radiographic image.

6. For pair production interactions:

$$E_i = 1.022 \; MeV + E_e + E_e+$$

$$2.5 \; MeV = 1.022 \; MeV + E_e + E_e+$$

$$E_e + E_e+ = 2.5 \; MeV - 1.022 \; MeV = 1.478 \; MeV$$

$$E_e = 0.60(1.478 \; MeV) \approx 0.8868 \; MeV \; or \; 886.8 \; keV$$

and

$$E_e+ = 1.478 \; MeV - 0.8868 \; MeV = 0.5912 \; MeV \; or \; 591.2 \; keV$$

7. A pair production event occurs in the vicinity of an atomic nucleus. Triplet production occurs in the vicinity of a shell electron.

8.

Given: $HVL = 1.3 \; mm \; Pb$

$$I_o = 120 \; mR$$

$$thickness = x = 3.5 \; mm \; Pb$$

$$I = ?$$

Using the attenuation equation,

$$I = I_o(0.5)^N$$

$$where \; N = \frac{x}{HVL} = \frac{3.5 \; mm \; Pb}{1.3 \; mm \; Pb} \approx 2.7$$

$$then \; I = (120 \; mR)(0.5)^{2.7}$$

$$= (120 \; mR)(0.154)$$

$$\approx 18.5 \; mR$$

9.   *Given*: I_o = 800 mR

                I = 620 mR

    thickness = x = 0.8 mm Al

           HVL = ?

From the attenuation equation,

$$I = I_o(0.5)^N$$

$$620 \text{ } mR = (800 \text{ } mR)(0.5)^N$$

$$(0.5)^N = \frac{620 \text{ } mR}{800 \text{ } mR} \approx 0.775$$

To solve for N, Take ln (or log) of both sides:

$$\ln(0.5)^N = \ln(0.775)$$

$$N \ln(0.5) = \ln 0.775$$

$$N(-0.693) = (-0.255)$$

$$N = \frac{-0.255}{-0.693} = 0.37$$

From definition, $N = \dfrac{x}{HVL}$ *or*

$$HVL = \frac{x}{N}$$

$$= \frac{0.8 \text{ } mm \text{ } Al}{0.37}$$

$$HVL \approx 2.2 \text{ } mm \text{ } Al$$

10.   *Given*: HVL = 2.2 mm Pb

             I_o = 950 mR

              I = 2 mR

    thickness = x = ?

Using the attenuation equation:

$$I = I_o(0.5)^N$$

$$2 \ mR = (950 \ mR)(0.5)^N$$

$$(0.5)^N = \frac{2 \ mR}{950 \ mR} \approx 0.002$$

To solve for N, take ln (or log) of both sides:

$$\ln(0.5)^N = \ln(0.002)$$

$$N \ln(0.5) = \ln 0.002$$

$$N(-0.693) \approx -6.215$$

$$N = \frac{-6.215}{-0.693} \approx 9$$

From definition of N,

$$N = \frac{x}{HVL}$$

or $\quad x = (N)(HVL)$

$$= (9)(2.2 \ mm \ Pb)$$

$$x \approx 19.8 \ mm \ Pb$$

11a. From the graph (see Figure 8-14), approximately 17.6% is transmitted by 2.5 HVLs.

  b. From the graph, 3.8 HVLs will *transmit* approximately 7.2%. Therefore the percent *attenuated* is 100% - 7.2% = 92.8%.

  c. From the graph, 30% *attenuated* represents 70% *transmitted*. 70% transmission corresponds to approximately 0.5 HVL. Therefore the thickness of Al needed is:

$$\text{thickness needed} = (0.5 \ HVL)(2.4 \ cm \ Al)$$

$$= 1.2 \ cm \ AL$$

  d. From the graph, 65% transmission corresponds to approximately 0.62 HVLs. Therefore the thickness of Pb needed will be:

$$\text{thickness needed} = (0.62 \ HVL)(0.6 \ mm \ Pb)$$

$$\approx 0.37 \ mm \ Pb$$

e. The percent transmission desired

$$\frac{20\ mR}{1200\ mR} \times 100\% = 1.7\%$$

From the graph, this corresponds to approximately 5.88 HVLs. Therefore the thickness needed:

thickness needed = (5.88 HVLs)(0.15 mm Pb)

$\approx$ 0.88 mm Pb

12. From HVL $\approx$ 3.1 mm Al; second HVL $\approx$ 4.8 mm Al

$$Homogeneity\ Coefficient \approx \frac{3.1}{4.8} \approx 0.65$$

Note: These are graphically determined values and may vary slightly from one graphical determination to another.

CHAPTER 9 SOLUTIONS

1. The x-ray emission spectrum is composed of all the x-rays emitted from the x-ray tube when the tube is activated. The spectrum includes both the bremsstrahlung and characteristic x-rays produced during tube operation.

2. The continuous spectrum is composed of all the x-rays produced by bremsstrahlung. These x-rays are produced as fast-moving electrons from the filament lose their energy through nonionizing interactions with target atoms.

   The discrete spectrum is composed of distinct energy characteristic x-rays. These characteristic x-rays arise when fast-moving electrons from the filament cause the ejection of inner-shell electrons of target atoms. As electrons from outer shells fall to fill in vacancies in the inner shells, characteristic x-rays are produced.

3. Energy shifts in the continuous spectrum are produced by changes in filtration, kVp, and voltage waveform used.

4. The number of x-rays in the continuous spectrum are affected by changes in filtration, kVp, mA, mAs, voltage waveform, distance to the x-ray source, and Z-number of the target.

5. Quantity (i.e., number of x-rays) of the discrete spectrum is affected by changes in the mA, mAs, kVp, filtration, distance to the x-ray source, Z-number of the target and the voltage waveform used.

6. Quality of the discrete spectrum is affected directly by changes in the Z-number of the target.

EXERCISE SOLUTIONS

1. a.
$$\lambda_{MIN} = \frac{12.4}{kVp}$$

$$= \frac{12.4}{60\ kVp} \approx 21\ \text{Å}$$

    b.
$$\lambda_{MIN} = \frac{12.4}{70\ kVp} \cong 0.18\ \text{Å}$$

    c.
$$\lambda_{MIN} = \frac{12.4}{80\ kVp} \cong 0.16\ \text{Å}$$

d. $\lambda_{MIN} = \dfrac{12.4}{90\ kVp} \cong 0.14\ \text{Å}$

e. $\lambda_{MIN} = \dfrac{12.4}{100\ kVp} \cong 0.12\ \text{Å}$

2. a. $\dfrac{I_1}{I_2} = \dfrac{(kVp_1)^2}{(kVp_2)^2}$

$\dfrac{110\ mR}{I_2} = \dfrac{(70\ kVp)^2}{(90\ kVp)^2}$

$\dfrac{110\ mR}{I_2} = \dfrac{4900}{8100} = \dfrac{49}{81}$

$(81)\ (110\ mR) = 49\ I_2$

$I_2 = \dfrac{(81)\ (110\ mR)}{49} \cong 181.8\ mR$

b. $\dfrac{110\ mR}{I_2} = \dfrac{(70\ kVp)^2}{(100\ kVp)^2}$

$\dfrac{110\ mR}{I_2} = \dfrac{4900}{10000} = \dfrac{49}{100}$

$49\ I_2 = (100)\ (110\ mR)$

$$I_2 = \frac{(100)\ (110\ mR)}{49} \cong 224.5\ mR$$

3.   a.

$$\frac{I_1}{I_2} = \frac{mAS_1}{mAS_2}$$

$$\frac{25\ mR}{I_2} = \frac{15\ mAS}{20\ mAS}$$

$$20\ (25\ mR) = (15)\ I_2$$

$$I_2 = \frac{20\ (25\ mR)}{15} \cong 33.3\ mR$$

b.

$$\frac{25\ mR}{I_2} = \frac{15\ mAS}{10\ mAS}$$

$$(15)\ (I_2) = (10)\ (25\ mR)$$

$$I_2 = \frac{10\ (25\ mR)}{15} \cong 16.7\ mR$$

4.   Given: $I_o = 100$ mR

        $I = 72$ mR

        Thickness = t = 1 mm AL

        HVL = ?

        $I = I_o\ (0.5)^N$

      $72\ mR = (100\ mR)\ (0.5)^N$

$$(0.5)^N = \frac{72 \; mR}{100 \; mR} = 0.72$$

To solve, take the natural log (ln) of both sides:

$$\ln (0.5)^N = \ln 0.72$$

$$N \ln (0.5) = \ln 0.72$$

$$N \; (-0.693) \cong (-0.33)$$

$$N = \frac{-0.33}{-0.693} \cong 0.48$$

but $N = \dfrac{t}{HVL}$, so:

$$\frac{t}{HVL} \cong 0.48$$

$$HVL = \frac{t}{0.48} = \frac{1 \; mm \; Al}{0.48} \cong 2.1 \; mm \; Al$$

5.

$$\frac{mAS_1}{mAS_2} = \left(\frac{d_1}{d_2}\right)^2$$

$$\frac{5}{x} = \left(\frac{40}{72}\right)^2$$

$$\frac{5}{x} = \frac{1600}{5184}$$

$$1600\ x\ =\ 25920$$

$$x\ =\ 16.2\ mAs$$

Note that if you take $(72)^2 \div (40)^2$, you can determine the multiplication factor needed to solve this problem, i.e., 3.24. Then $5 \times 3.24 = 16.2$. The most common distances used are 40" and 72". In a pinch, when unable to calculate exact mAs changes due to distance, note that there is a relationship of ~ 3 between 72" and 40". Thus if moving from 40" to 72", increase mAs by a factor of 3; from 72" to 40", divide mAs by 3.

CHAPTER 10 SOLUTIONS

1. Glass.

2. Strong, can be made thin and does not ignite during storage.

3. Maintains silver bromide in suspension, can be made hard and remain porous, and permits swelling and shrinking to retain the silver.

4. Silver bromide suspended in gelatin.

5. Upon exposure to radiation the crystals absorb the energy and electrons are emitted or move from their normal orbital position and travel at random throughout the crystal. Some will be trapped by the speck making the speck electrically charged. The speck now being negatively charged will cause positive ions to gravitate to the speck. Here they unite and neutralize forming atoms of metallic silver. As more silver ions are neutralized the speck grows in size in response to the amount of radiation energy absorbed. This

physical change produces the latent image.

6. Density of a radiograph is the amount of metallic silver distributed on the film.

7. The radiation exposure required to produce a specific density is a measure of film sensitivity.

8. Sensitivity and latitude

9. Latitude is the film's ability to display many shades of gray ranging from light to black. Contrast is a variation in density.

10. To reduce patient exposure and prevent overloading equipment

11. Developer, fixer, wash and drying

12. Hydroquinone and metol or phenidone

13. Thiosulfate

14. To aid in the prevention of ionization

15. Higher temperature and higher concentration of solutions

CHAPTER 11 SOLUTIONS

1. Definitions:

   a. A **radiograph** is the image of an object produced when x-rays pass through the object, forming a pattern of radiant energies which emerge from the object and are recorded and become visible after chemical processing of the image receptor (film).

   b. **Radiography** is the production of an image by passing x-rays through an object and intercepting the energy emerging from the object with a sensitive emulsion.

   c. A **radiographer** is a person educated in the art and science of radiography to become qualified to produce images of objects by passing x-rays through the object, recording the pattern of radiant energy emerging from the object, and processing the image receptor (film).

d. The **background density** of a radiographic image occurs in the areas where no object part is interposed between the x-ray source and the film producing blackening about the outer borders of the image.

e. **Elongation** is a form of distortion. It exists if the image demonstrates the object as longer than it actually is or a specific part of the object appears longer in relation to other parts in the image.

f. **Magnification** is a misrepresentation of the size of the object in the image, making it appear larger than expected in proportion to surrounding structures.

g. A **latent image** is an invisible image formed by ionized silver halide crystals of the emulsion layer of the film. This ionization is produced by the absorption of an x-ray photon pattern formed by passage through an object.

h. **Preliminary radiographs** are images to visualize the plain anatomy of the part. These are made early in a radiographic procedure before any changes are made which will alter or obscure visualization of the natural anatomy.

i. **Remnant radiation** is all of the x-radiation emerging from an object to reach the film and produce an image in its sensitive emulsion.

j. **Fog** is an unwanted density which is spread evenly over the image, giving it a hazy, darker appearance.

k.   The term **penetrability** refers to a property of a material which indicates how easily something (in this case x-radiation) can pass through the material.

l.   The **radiation intensity** refers to the quantity of x-rays existent in a specified area.

m.   A **requisition** is a request for radiologic consultation. Usually, this consists of a form that is completed by the referring physician to signify a request for a radiographic procedure of a particular patient to be performed and interpreted by a radiologist.

n.   An **x-ray** is an electromagnetic energy form. In diagnostic radiography, x-rays usually have a wavelength between 0.1 A and 0.5 A.

o.   **Radiopaque** refers to a property of a material which resists the passage of x-rays through it; i.e., the material absorbs most of the radiation which is incident upon it.

p.   **Radiolucent** refers to a property of a material which offers very little hindrance to the passage of x-rays; i.e., the material absorbs only a small amount of the radiation incident upon it.

2. The four (4) radiographic qualities identified in this chapter were:

Radiographic density is the overall blackening of the radiographic image.

Radiographic contrast refers to the difference between adjacent densities (grays) within the radiographic image.

74

This quality consists of two parts:

Film contrast is the inherent property of a film which allows differences in densities to be recorded as a result of the medical x-ray film manufacturing process and the chemical development process.

Subject contrast is the result of variations in absorption of x-radiation by the different tissues of the body.

Radiographic detail refers to the structural fine lines of parts as represented in a radiographic image.

Radiographic distortion is the misrepresentation of the object in its image. There are two types:

Misrepresentation of shape in which the image outline(s) of an object or part is misrepresented, i.e., elongated or foreshortened.

Misrepresentation of size in which the area measurements of a structure in its image differ from those of the structure. The image measurements are larger; therefore, this is referred to as magnification.

3. The radiographic qualities of radiographic density, radiographic contrast, and image sharpness are closely related because of their interdependence on each other.

Radiographic density is the darkening of the film produced by

75

deposits of black metallic silver to form the image. This quality is dependent upon sufficient penetration of the x-rays to produce these deposits.

The radiographic contrast is the pattern of deposit of the black metallic silver that forms the image and infers differences in the amount deposited in the various areas of the image. This quality is dependent on the presence of adequate radiographic density for its demonstration and upon the degree of penetration of the part.

Radiographic detail is a term referring to the image sharpness of the structures appearing in the image, i.e., clear distinct outlining of the structure of the parts in the image. This quality is dependent upon radiographic contrast for visualization.

4. Differentiations:

    a. Film contrast is the inherent difference in adjacent image densities as a result of the film manufacturing procedure and chemical processing of the image. Subject contrast is object dependent. That is, it depends on the absorption characteristics of the material composition of the object that is imaged.

    b. A "long scale of contrast in an image" means that a large number of density shades (grays) are represented in the image.
        A "short scale of contrast in an image" exists if a small number of density shades are represented in the image.

c. A "high contrast image" is one in which there is a large
    percentage difference between the density shades within
    it.
    A "low contrast image" is one in which the percentage
    difference between the density shades is small.
d. Primary radiation is the radiation from the source
    which retains its original energy and direction.

    Scatter radiation refers to primary radiation which has
    undergone change(s) in energy, direction, or both.
    Secondary radiation is often included in this term
    because it is primary radiation which has experienced
    changes.

    Remnant radiation is the radiation which emerges from
    the object to expose a sensitive emulsion (film) and form
    an image.

5. Relationships:
a. Radiographic density and mAs are directly proportional to
    each other. As the mAs is increased or decreased, the
    radiographic density increases or decreases in the same
    proportion; i.e., if mAs is doubled, the radiographic
    density will be doubled.
b. For purposes of maintaining a given average density of a
    radiographic image, the mAs is directly proportional to
    the source-image distance (SID) squared.
    The formula here for calculating the new mAs to be used
    for changes in SID from that normally required for the

77

part to be radiographed is:

$$\frac{mAs_1}{SID_1^2} = \frac{mAs_2}{SID_2^2}$$

What this means in general is that as the SID increases the mAs must also be increased. This is true because the amount of x-radiation which reaches any particular unit area decreases.

This relationship exists because x-rays are emitted at all angles from their source and travel in straight lines from that source. An example is outlined below to better explain this phenomena.

If the mAs and SID used for a particular exposure produce a specific density on a 10" x 12" (120 square inches) film at an SID of 36" and the SID is increased to 72". The radiation traveling in straight lines from the source diverges and the same amount of radiation is distributed over an area 20" x 24" (480 square inches; four times the original area). This means that the number of x-ray photons to each unit area of the film is now one-fourth of what it was originally because the original quantity of photons is the same. In order to ensure the same number of photons will reach the 10" x 12" film the primary radiation must be increased by a factor of 4. Assume that the original exposure deposited 100 photons per square inch. That means there were 12,000 total photons deposited on the original exposure at 36". At 72", these same 12,000 photons will be dispersed over an area of 480 square inches, or approximately 25 photons per square inch if the source is not increased. To bring the number of photons per square inch back to 100, 4 times as many photons must be produced.

A simple way of expressing this would be to say that the mAs change necessary to obtain the radiographic density required when the SID is changed is equal to the square of the ratio of the new SID to the original SID multiplied by the original mAs. The formula for this would be:

$$mAs_2 = \left(\frac{SID_2}{SID_1}\right)^2 \times mAs_1$$

Use of this formula will permit compensation for radiographic density when the source-image distance is altered for an exposure.

c. For purposes of maintaining a given density, the mA is inversely proportional to the exposure time. In order to produce the same density, the mAs must remain constant. This means that as mA is increased, the exposure time, s, must be decreased by the reciprocal of the amount the mA change.

d. To maintain a given density, the mAs can be compensated for by changing the kVP for the exposure. The rule is, for a given density if the mAs is halved, the kVp must be increased by 15% at any kVp level to maintain a constant average density of the image. This is an inverse relationship, but the amount of change of one factor is not the reciprocal of the change in the other.

6. Three simple methods of doubling the radiographic image density from the control panel of the x-ray machine are:

   a.   Increase the kVp by 15%; i.e., $kVp_1 + .15kVp_1 = kVp_2$, or

   b.   Double the mA used for the original exposure, or

   c.   Double the exposure time used for the original exposure.

7. Exposure factors that produce an image with a satisfactory density level can be altered to produce images with a different contrast scale. If a longer scale is required, the changes should effect an increase of the x-ray penetration factor, kVp, and a decrease of the radiographic density factor, mAs. If a shorter scale is desired, the kVp would be decreased with an increase in the mAs that is indicated by the relationship statement.

Take the original exposure factors for the image in which the contrast scale is to be lengthened. Keep all factors as they were except the kVp and mAs. Then perform the following in the order given:

   a.   Increase the kVp by 15%.

   b.   Half the original mAs

        (half the exposure time or the mA but not both).

   c.   Expose the film.

   d.   Process the film.

   e.   Inspect the image for satisfactory change.

If the contrast level is the desired one, stop the process. If it is not, continue the process using the exposure factors from the immediate past image. Keep in mind that larger changes are gained by adding 15% to the kVp and halving the mAs; smaller changes are effected by easing the kVp by 5% and decreasing the mAs by 30%, or one-third.

8. The method used to calculate the minimum kVp to penetrate any part for radiography depends on the type generator used to supply the electric current for machine operation. For single-phase generation, double the centimeter measurement of the part and add the constant 30 to obtain the minimum kVp to penetrate the part. Three-phase generation requires doubling the part's centimeter measurement and adding the constant 25 to that number to yield the minimum kilovoltage to penetrate the part.

9. The minimum kVp for part penetration is seldom used in modern radiology departments because the higher mAs value is required for these exposures. This gives a higher contrast image than most radiologists prefer and the radiation dosage absorbed by the patient is greater than necessary.

10. An exposure technique chart is a guide to the exposure factors and conditions used to demonstrate a particular anatomical part of a patient.

It is used by measuring the part along the path of the beam's central ray. Take that measurement to the chart and then:
Locate the part to be radiographed.

Locate the projection to be performed.

Find the centimeter measurement of the part in the part-projection section of the chart.

In adjacent lines or columns will be the mAs and kVp to be used for the exposure.

Establish the mAs and kVp specified by the chart at the machine's control panel.

Ensure all other exposure requirements are applied.

Make minor adjustments in kVp or mAs that are made necessary by pathology or other conditions present.

11. a.   The primary radiographic exposure factors are:
Kilovoltage refers to 1000 volt increments.
The kilovolt is the unit of measure of the tube voltage that determines the kinetic energy of the electrons flowing in the x-ray tube to produce x-rays.
kV is its abbreviation.

kVp is the abbreviation for peak kilovoltage which determines the maximum energy of an electron in the electron stream. This maximum energy defines the minimum wavelength in the x-ray beam.

Milliamperage refers to the quantity of electrons flowing past a point between the cathode and anode of the x-ray tube in a single unit of time. It is a measure of tube current.

Exposure time is the length of time that electrons are

allowed to flow in the x-ray tube during an exposure. The time units used in x-ray photon production are seconds (*s*) and milliseconds (*ms*).

Milliampere-seconds is a value indicating the total quantity of electrons flowing through an x-ray tube during an x-ray exposure. It is a product of the number electrons flowing per unit of time and the length of time they flow. mAs is the abbreviation used.

Source-image distance (SID) is the distance from the source (x-ray tube anode) to the image receptor expressed in units of inches or centimeters.

  b. The penetration of the part by the x-rays in the beam are controlled by the kilovoltage (kV) used to produce the beam. Higher kilovoltage produces a more penetrating beam.

  c. A predictable quantitative effect on radiographic density is produced by (1) the combination of the mA and exposure time or (2) the SID used for the exposure.

It is preferable to change the mAs to alter the image density. This combination directly effects the number of x-rays produced. A change in the SID alters other qualities as well as radiographic density.

Example:

The exposure factors obtained from the technique chart for a particular projection are:

```
        400 speed screen                     62 kVp

        Bucky, 12:1 grid                      6.66 mAs

        11 cm measurement of body part        40" SID
```

The image requires that the radiographic density be
doubled. There are two ways to do this without changing
kVp (penetration and contrast scale). The most preferable
way is to double the mAs (from 6.66 mAs to 13.32 mAs can
be accomplished by using 200 mA at 1/15 second or 100 mAs
at 2/15 second instead of 100 mAs at 1/15 second. The
radiographic density will be doubled, the radiographic
contrast will be the same, and the radiographic detail
suffers insignificant detriment.

The second way to double the density would be to reduce
the SID from 40" to about 28.3". The radiographic
density will be doubled, the radiographic contrast
will remain the same, but the radiographic detail is
decreased significantly and the magnification of the
object in the image is increased.

12. To produce images of the anatomic parts of the human body the
    x-ray beam from the source passes through the anatomical part
    to the image receptor. The beam is composed of x-rays of
    different wavelengths capable of different degrees of
    penetration. The part is composed of various tissues of
    different absorption characteristics. The x-rays interact
    with the tissues. The parts with higher atomic number and

electron density absorb most of the x-rays which try to pass through them, thus creating bright images of these structures. Other x-rays are only partially absorbed by the tissues they attempt to pass through and create images of varying gray intensities. The easily penetrated structures form darker images than those which are harder to penetrate. X-rays pass through these structures readily without being absorbed. These produce a very dark or black shadow within the image.

13. Combinations of mA and exposure time to yield a radiographic density equal to that produced by 15 mAs.

Possible mA values available: 100 mA, 200 mA, 400 mA, 600 mA, 800 mA, 1000 mA, and 1200 mA.

The machine has a three-phase generator.

The exposure times are expressed as fractions and as decimals.

a. 100 mA

15 mAs/100 mA

0.15 or 3/20 sec

b. 200 mA

15 mAs/200 mA

0.075 or 3/40 sec

c. 400 mA

15 mAs/400 mA

0.0375 or 3/80 sec

d. 600 mA

15 mAs/600 mA

0.025 or 1/40 sec

e. 800 ma

15 mAs/800 mA

0.01875 or 3/160 sec

f. 1000 mA

15 mAs/1000 mA

0.015 or 3/200 sec

g. 1200 mA

15 mAs/1200 mA

.0125 or 1/80 sec

Three-phase, 6-pulse current (from the physics chapters) supplies 360 impulses of current each second; three-phase, 12-pulse current supplies 720 impulses per second. The exposure times selected to adequately supply the current for the exposure with these mA values must be evenly divisible by

360 (or 720) or can be divided into 360 (or 720) evenly.

If the current is three-phase, 6-pulse, a., b., c., d., e., and g. comply with this determinant; f. is the only one which does not. If three-phase, 12-pulse current, all (a. - g.) may be used.

14. A lateral cervical spine should be produced using the exposure factors 65 mAs, 70 kVp, and 72" SID with a grid. The same projection of the cervical spine must be performed using the same grid at an SID of 40". If the kVp remains at 70, the mAs must be changed.

The mAs must be decreased because the SID will be decreased. Use the rule, the mAs used for an exposure to produce the same radiographic density is directly proportional to the SID squared.

In this case, the new mAs will be found by setting it equal to the ratio of the new SID to the original SID (40"/72") squared times the original mAs.

$$mAs_2 = \left(\frac{SID_2}{SID_1} \right)^2 \times mAs_1$$

$$mAs_2 = \left(\frac{40''}{72''} \right)^2 \times 65 \ mAs$$

$$= \left(\frac{5}{9} \right)^2 \times 65 \ mAs$$

$$= \left(\frac{25}{81} \right) \times 65 \ mAs$$

$$mAs_2 = 20.06 \ or \ 20 \ mAs$$

15. The mA and exposure time combinations that must be used to radiograph the lateral cervical spine in question number 14 if the mA values available are 50, 100, 200, 300, 500 and 600 with a single-phase unit are:

Single phase current (from the physics chapters) supplies 120 impulses of current each second. The exposure times selected to adequately supply the current for the exposure with these mA values must be evenly divisible by 120 or can be divided into 120 evenly.

a. 50 mA

   20 mAs/50 mA

    0.4 or 2/5 sec

b. 100 mA

   20 mAs/100 mA

    0.2 or 1/5 sec

c. 200 mA

   20 mAs/200 mA

    0.1 or 1/10 sec

d. 300

   20 mAs/300 mA

   0.067 or 1/15 sec

e. 500

   20 mAs/500 mA

   0.04 or 1/25 sec

f. 600

   20 mAs/600mA

   0.033 or 1/30 sec

All mA and time combinations will work with the single phase machine except e.

16. The normal radiograph of the hand per the technique chart requires:

400 Speed of S/F combination   40" SID   Nongrid

cm	2	3	4	5	6	7	8
kV	58	58	58	58	60	63	66
mAs	1.15	1.35	1.52	1.89	1.90	2.01	2.03

The hand measures 4 cm in the anteroposterior direction.
Therefore the kVp and mAs to use would be 58 kVp and 1.52 mAs.
In order to shorten the contrast scale the mAs must increased
and the kVp lowered. The reverse of the rule that states that
for a given image density the kVp may be increased by 15% if
the mAs halved (refer to this rule in the text if needed). If
the mAs is doubled you decrease the kVp by ~13%.

Multiply the mAs x 2:   1.52 x 2 = 3.04 mAs

Lower the kVp by 13%:   58 - 0.13(58) =

58 - 7.54 = 50.46 kVp

The calculated kVp_{min} to penetrate a hand of this size is:

(2 x 4) + 30 (single phase equipment) = 38 kVp

or (2 x 4) + 25 (three phase equipment) = 33 kVp

At the 50.46 kVp calculated for the shorter contrast
projection of the 4 cm hand, the radiographer does not have to
be concerned about not penetrating the part.

17. a. The mAs value derived in question 16 can be obtained
with the mA values and machine in question 15 by using:

a. 3 mAs/ 50 mA = 0.06 or 3/50 sec   Will not work

b. 3 mAs/ 100 mA = 0.03 or 3/100 sec   Will not work

c. 3 mAs/ 200 mA = 0.015 or 3/200 sec   Will not work

d. 3 mAs/ 300 mA = 0.001 or 1/100 sec   Will not work

e. 3 mAs/ 500 mA = 0.006 or 3/500 sec   Will not work

f. 3 mAs/ 600 mA = 0.005 or 1/200 sec   Will not work

This machine does not have a combination of mA and exposure time that will yield exactly 3 mAs.

b.   The mA given for the machine in question 13 that can be used to give the mAs value derived in question 16 is:

Three-phase, 6-pulse current:

a. 3 mAs/ 100 mA = 0.03 or 3/100 sec   Will not work

b. 3 mAs/ 200 mA = 0.015 or 3/200 sec   Will not work

c. 3 mAs/ 400 mA = 0.0075 or 3/400 sec   Will not work

d. 3 mAs/ 600 mA = 0.005 or 1/200 sec   Will not work

e. 3 mAs/ 800 mA = 0.00375 or 3/800 sec   Will not work

f. 3 mAs/ 1000 mA = 0.003 or 3/1000 sec   Will not work

g. 3 mAs/ 1200 mA = 0.0025 or 1/400 sec   Will not work

None of these combinations of mA and exposure time will yield exactly 3 mAs.

These calculations were followed for three-phase, 12 pulse current and again there were no combinations which yielded exactly 3 mAs.

Further changes in exposure factors were made of increasing the mAs by 30% and decreasing the kVp by 5%. This brought the exposure factors to 4 mAs and 48 kVp.

Again, no combination of exposure time and mA could be found that yielded exactly 4 mAs. All current type machines were checked mathematically.

If this mAs is increased by 30% and this kVp is decreased by 5% one more time, the exposure time - mA combinations which will work are:

5 of the possible 6 combinations with single-phase equipment; 2 of the possible 7 combinations with three-phase, 6-pulse equipment; and 4 of the possible 7 combinations with three-phase, 12-pulse equipment.

The kVp levels above the calculated minimum kVp can be maintained with the combinations that can be used.

CHAPTER 12 SOLUTIONS

1. Photographic properties include the factors of density and contrast. Density refers to the overall blackness represented on a radiographic image. Contrast refers to the difference in adjacent densities on a radiograph. Photographic properties refer to visibility of structural details on a radiographic image while geometric properties refer to the sharpness of structural details on a radiograph. Detail and distortion are known as geometric properties. Detail can be defined as how one an visualize fine line structural edges on a radiograph.

Distortion refers to the mispresentation of the size and shape of an object on the radiographic image.

2. An image of satisfactory radiographic quality must have a proper balance between visibility and sharpness of detail. An image must possess proper density, sufficient contrast, maximum detail and minimum distortion in order to be considered a satisfactory radiograph. An image containing proper density and contrast is of little value if the structural details are unsharp.

3. The use of a faster film/screen combination would be the first choice. This will allow the use of a shorter exposure time, resulting in less radiation dose to the patient since the milliampere-seconds (MAS) would be decreased.

4. Decreasing SID will increase distortion of the radiographic image. This is usually a result of magnification; as SID is decreased magnification increases which results in a decrease in overall detail of the radiographic image.

5. Image resolution is also known as detail and can be be defined as how well fine line structures are seen radiographically. Resolution can be determined by the number of line pairs per millimeter that the imaging system is capable of recording. Resolution of the image can be identified by testing the image with a device known as a resolution grid.

6.

$$MAGNIFICATION = \frac{Image\ Width}{Object\ Width}$$

or

$$MAGNIFICATION = \frac{SID}{SID-OFD}$$

7.

$$PERCENTAGE\ OF\ MAGNIFICATION = \frac{IW-OW}{OW} \times 100$$

or

$$PERCENTAGE\ OF\ MAGNIFICATION = \frac{SID-*SOD}{*SOD} \times 100$$

*SOD = SID - OFD

8. As SID increases radiation intensity decreases according to the inverse square law. Therefore, in order to maintain a satisfactory density level the milliampere-seconds (MAS) will need to be increased. To accomplish this the milliamperage (mA) and the exposure time must be increased. Whenever there is an increase in exposure time, there is always the possiblity of motion unsharpness due to patient movement or breathing during the radiographic exposure.

9. As screen speed increases radiographic detail decreases and vice versa. The amount of loss of detail depends on the screen/film combination used and their resolution properties. High speed - low resolution screens are useful when radiation dose must be kept to a minimum and exposure time very short, however, low speed screens provide the best radiographic detail.

10. Yes. Because in order to have a proper balance of geometric properties the radiograph must possess maximum detail and minimum distortion. In order to have sharppness of structural

details, the visibility of structural details must also be properly balanced. This is accomplished by the use of adequate density and contrast. The preceding statements are true provided there is no motion unsharpness or screen unsharpness present on the radiographic image.

11. First a diagram must be constructed to determine the width of the image, then apply proportions.

$$\frac{image\ width}{Object\ width} = \frac{SID}{SID\text{-}OFD}$$

$$\frac{image\ width}{12\ in.} = \frac{40\ in.}{40\ in.\ -\ 10\ in.}$$

$$\frac{image\ width}{12\ in.} = \frac{40\ in.}{30\ in.}$$

$$image\ width = \frac{40 \times 12}{30} = \frac{480}{30} = 16\ in.$$

a.

$$MAGNIFICATION\ FACTOR = \frac{image\ width}{object\ width} = \frac{16}{12} = 1.33$$

b.

$$PERCENTAGE\ OF\ MAGNIFICATION = \frac{image\ width\text{-}object\ width}{object\ width} \times 100$$

$$= \frac{16-12}{12} \times 100$$

$$= .33 \times 100 = 33.3\%$$

CHAPTER 13 SOLUTIONS

1.   The **anode heel effect** refers to a variation in the
       intensity of an x-ray beam long the longitudinal axis of
       the x-ray tube. The beam is less intense at the anode
       end of the beam because more of the x-rays produced at
       the anode must travel through the anode to escape the
       tube. Therefore more of these x-rays are absorbed than
       at the cathode end of the x-ray beam.

2.   The **result of the anode heel effect** in the radiographic
       image is the radiographic density of the radiograph is
       diminished toward the anode end of the beam. This is
       especially true if the part requires a large or long
       radiation field and is radiographed at a shorter
       source-image distance (40" SID or less).

3.   An **x-ray beam filter** is a sheet of metal which is placed
       in the x-ray beam before it reaches the patient.

4.   The **purpose of a filter in the x-ray beam** is to absorb
       the longer wavelengths (lower energy) in the x-ray beam
       before it reaches the patient. These longer x-ray
       wavelengths are those which would be absorbed by the
       patient without contributing anything to the radiographic
       image.

5.   The **amount of x-ray beam filtration** is usually **expressed**
       as mm of aluminum or as mm of aluminum equivalent. It is
       expressed in this manner because the filter normally used
       in diagnostic radiography is composed of aluminum.

6. Definitions:

   a.   **Added filtration** is a thickness of a stated metal which is inserted into the x-ray beam external to the x-ray tube.

b.   **Inherent filtration** consists of parts of the tube and tube housing which absorb some of the lower energy photon radiation, thus forming a natural filtration of the x-ray beam as a result of the construction and support mechanisms of the x-ray tube. This filtration is expressed in mm of aluminum equivalent.

c.   The **total filtration** of an x-ray beam is the total of the inherent filtration and the added filtration in the x-ray beam emerging from an x-ray tube.

d.   A **compensating filter** is a material which is placed in the x-ray beam to provide an image of sufficient overall density even though the anatomical part varies in density or thickness. The filter is used over the thinner or less dense areas while the normal beam from the x-ray tube records the thicker or denser portion(s) of the anatomical part.

7. a.   For an **x-ray beam whose kVp is less than 50 kVp,** the total filtration of the beam must be a minimum of 0.5 mm of Al or Al equivalence.

b.   For an **x-ray beam whose kVp is between 50 kVp and 70 kVp,** the total filtration of the beam must be a minimum of 1.5 mm of Al or Al equivalence.

c.   For **an x-ray beam whose kVp is greater than 70 kVp,** the total filtration of the beam must be a minimum of 2.5 mm of Al or Al equivalence.

8. A **filter in the x-ray beam** removes the lower energy

photons from the beam before it reaches the patient. These lower energy x-rays would be absorbed by the patient and contribute to the patient's absorbed radiation dosage.

9. A **beam restrictor** is used in an x-ray beam to limit the size of the x-ray beam as it exits the x-ray tube area and before it reaches the patient.

10. A **diaphragm** is a device consisting of a small metal sheet or plate of an x-ray absorbent metal with an aperture in its center for the passage of a particular portion of the x-ray beam.

A **cylinder cone** is a device consisting of a metal cylinder, which may or may not be slightly flared at the end away from the x-ray tube, mounted to a base. The base may be described as a diaphragm. The effective aperture of this device is the end of the cylinder which is nearer the patient.

An **extension cylinder cone** is a special type of cylinder cone. This device has, in addition to the metal cylinder and the base, a second cylinder outside the one that attaches to the base. This second cylinder acts as a sleeve which can be extended to bring the aperture to a point even closer to the patient.

A **collimator** is a device which is permanently mounted to the lower portion of the x-ray tube housing. The collimator is equipped with two sets of leaded shutters, one nearer the x-ray tube and the other more distal from the tube. Each set of shutters forms an aperture that permits the passage of the central portion of the x-ray beam through it. The aperture away from the tube is larger than the one nearer the tube. The size of each aperture is adjusted by moving four shutters, two regulate the beam laterally and two regulate the beam longitudinally.

12. a. **Diaphragms**

Advantages: Restricts the size of the x-ray beam. Two shapes are generally available.

Disadvantages: Physical interchange of diaphragms is required to limit the beam size to the part size. Adjustment for various part sizes requires a large number present in each radiographic room. Rim of aperture may produce secondary radiation which will reach and be absorbed by the patient.

b. **Cylinder cones**

Advantages: Restricts the size of the x-ray beam. Much of the secondary radiation from the rim of the initial beam limiting aperture at the base of the cone is removed from the beam. The effective beam limiting aperture is closer to the patient. Two shapes are generally available, although the circular shape is more common.

Disadvantages: Physical interchange of cones is required to limit the beam size to the part size.

Adjustment for various sizes requires a
large number present in the radiographic
room. Devices, because of construction,
occupy more space in the radiographic room
and are heavier than diaphragms which
requires more exertion during the
interchange of devices.

c. **Extension cylinder cones**

Advantages: Much the same as are listed for cylinder
cones. Reduces beam for very small parts
because aperture can be brought into close
proximity to the part (T-M joints, mastoids,
gall bladder, or spot films of individual
vertebrae, etc.)

Disadvantages: Limited to use of particular parts, i.e.,
very small parts. Weight involved during
interchange, or currently during
attachment, is excessive.

d. **Collimator**

Advantages: Secondary radiation from the aperture rim
nearest the patient is much less. Aperture
size is easily adjusted to size of the part.
Presents a light localizer in collimator. Size
of light field coincides with radiation field
size, crosshair on lower surface of the
collimator which indicates the position of the
central beam of the x-ray field, and lighting
necessary to properly center the Bucky to the

radiant beam.

Disadvantages: Malfunction of the parts listed under "advantages" inconvenience equipment operators. The majority are limited to a beam shape which is rectangular.

13. Beam restrictors were developed to limit the radiation exposure of those persons undergoing radiographic or therapeutic procedures by limiting the area exposed to radiation to the size of the part of interest.

14. The **effect of the beam restrictor in radiography** is a reduction in the overall density of a radiographic image and an increase in the differences between the densities (radiographic contrast). Together these changes enable better visibility of image sharpness of the structures radiographed.

The beam restrictor accomplishes this because, in limiting the area exposed, it also limits the volume of tissue that can produce radiographically effective secondary radiation. This secondary radiation produces an overall haze of increased density in the radiographic image. If the production of the secondary radiation is limited, less reaches the film and the effects mentioned earlier that improve the quality of the mage occur.

15. a. When the **beam restriction is increased,** a radiographer should increase the exposure factors. The decision will be determined by the three factors which govern the production of secondary radiation. These

factors are:

(1) the volume of the part exposed. In this case, what is the degree of change in the volume of tissue exposed should be asked; (2) the density of the tissue exposed. The correct answer to does the volume to be radiographically exposed contain a large amount of air, fluid or muscle, bone, etc. should be determined. (3) the kilovoltage used for the exposure of the tissue volume. After considering these factors, the radiographer should correctly conclude whether to increase the exposure factors or not.

b. If the **beam restriction is decreased**, generally the radiographer should decrease the exposure factors. Before deciding to do this each radiographer should go through the same mental exercise given in the answer to "5. a.".

16. **Positive beam limitation (PBL)** is a system, now incorporated into all radiographic equipment, which produces automatic control of the collimation to the film size used for any radiograph produced using a cassette with film in a special holder (Bucky tray for example).

17. The **purpose of PBL** is to ensure that equipment operators will limit the area of the patient exposed to the area visualized in the image produced by that radiation exposure.

18. When the radiographic equipment incorporates a PBL, cassettes or film holders must be placed and locked into

a special holder. This special holder senses the film size and relays this information to the collimator, which must be adjusted to an aperture that allows a maximum beam size to permit the particular film to be exposed.

Exposures requiring table-top exposure techniques may not benefit from this equipment requirement. Some examples are mobile radiography, extremity radiography, etc.

19. a. A higher screen speed increases the **radiographic density** produced at given exposure factors. If the screen speed is lower, the radiographic density decreases for the same exposure.

   b. **Radiographic contrast** increases as the screen speed increases and appears to decrease as the screen speed decreases for a specific set of exposure factors.

   c. As the screen speed increases, the **production of image sharpness** decreases; as the screen speed decreases it is possible to increase the image sharpness produced in the image.

   d. It is possible to reduce exposure factors if a higher speed screen is used. By reducing the exposure factors there is less radiation to be **absorbed** if the exposure factor is not the kVp factor. If the kVp factor is the one reduced the absorption of radiation may be increased. For a lower screen speed the exposure factors may be increased thereby increasing the radiation to be absorbed. If the kVp factor is the exposure factor increased, more of the radiation produced will penetrate the part and the amount of radiation absorbed may actually decrease.

    e. Screen speed depends to a large extent upon the ability of the phosphor crystal layer to **convert the x-ray photon energy to light energy**. As the conversion efficiency of the phosphor compound used increases the screen speed increases. Conversely as the phosphor compound's conversion efficiency decreases the screen speed decreases.

20. An **intensifying screen** is a device developed to increase the effect of an x-ray exposure on the medical x-ray film to form an image.

21. a. The factors in radiography that should be considered which alter the **production of scatter radiation are:**

      (1) The kVp used to produce the image. As the kilovoltage level of the beam increases, more scatter radiation reaches the film.

      (2) The volume of the tissue to be irradiated with each part radiographed. In general, as the volume of tissue increases the amount of secondary radiation will increase. Before any decision regarding ume of tissue is made, part "3" of this answer must be considered. The volume of tissue is governed by the area irradiated and the thickness of the area.

      (3) The type of tissue in the irradiated volume. Is the volume of tissue air-filled (normally or abnormally)? Does it contain a large percentage of

bone? Is there a large amount of fluid or muscle present in the volume (normally or abnormally)? These are all the questions which need consideration.

b. The production on scattered radiation may be reduced by (following the outline established in "a" above),

(1) If the kVp is reduced to decrease the production of radiographically effective secondary radiation, the secondary radiation may still be produced but absorbed by the patient before it emerges to contribute radiographic density in the image.

(2) The volume of tissue irradiated can be decreased to reduce the production of secondary radiation. The first thing to do to decrease the volume irradiated is reduce the size of the aperture of the beam restrictor. This reduces the area irradiated and therefore the volume of tissue. If necessary, application of some contact lead shielding between the tube and the patient can be used to further shape and limit the volume irradiated. Decreasing the volume of tissue may require an increase in the exposure factors to restore the radiographic density level of the image.

The part thickness can be decreased by compression devices. These should be applied in the direction of beam travel through the part. If the thickness is decreased, the volume through which the beam must travel is reduced.

(3) There is not too much that can be done about the type tissue in the part to be radiographed except those things mentioned in "(1)" and "(2)" above. The radiographer does need to be aware of the type tissue and its potential to produce more or less radiographically effective secondary radiation as a result of the its normal anatomy or any pathologic or traumatic conditions in the area of interest.

22. **"Fog"** in radiography refers to an unwanted density covering the image and obscuring details in that image. Fog appears as a gray haze covering the image. The shade of added gray depends on the amount of exposure received that is not needed.

23. Those items which **reduce or can reduce the radiation dose of the patient** included:

a. Kilovoltage used to produce the images: This exposure factor controls the energy of the x-ray photons in the beam. If the kVp is increased, the beam's average energy increases and the beam becomes more penetrating. More x-ray photons exit the patient unchanged. If kV is increased the mAs should be decreased to maintain the image density. This means fewer x-ray photons are produced to be absorbed.

b. Filtration (added and inherent) absorbs the lower energy x-ray photons. This absorption reduces the number of the x-ray photons that are easily absorbed by the patient. Filters consist of thickness of a stated metal

104

(usually aluminum in diagnostic radiography) or other
material (stated in mm of Al equivalency) in the x-ray
beam which absorb low energy x-ray photons. The total
filtration used for most radiographic exposures is
2.5 mm of aluminum. If more is added to the beam there
is very little benefit realized from the addition.

c. Beam restrictor is a device to limit the size of the
x-ray beam to the area of radiographic interest. This
reduces the volume of the patient's tissue exposed to
radiation and therefore limits absorption of radiation
by the patient.

d. Intensifying screens are devices used in radiography to
convert x-ray energy to a light energy to which the
image receptor (sensitive film emulsion) is more
sensitive than it is to x-ray energy. Use of these
allows radiographic exposures to be decreased which also
reduces the radiation absorbed by the patient because
less radiation is available to absorb.

24. **Calcium tungstate intensifying screens** are used in
radiography to increase the effect of the radiation in the
radiographic image. The calcium tungstate phosphors of the
screen absorb about 20% of the x-rays incident upon them.
The efficiency with which this phosphor converts x-ray energy
to light energy is about 5%.

Rare earth intensifying screens fulfill the same purpose,
however these absorb about 40% to 60% of the incident x-ray
photons and convert about 20% of that to light. Therefore,

for a given x-ray exposure, the rare earth intensifying screens will provide much more ligh to effect the emulsion of the film.

25. Direct x-ray exposure of the medical x-ray film to produce an image of an anatomical part is about 32 times higher than would be required to produce the same image with a particular speed screen (X-Omatic Fine). This screen represents the maximum exposure that would be needed by an intensifying screen, 1/32 of the nonscreen exposure. Other intensifying screens require even less. The smallest exposure currently available is about 1/1200 of the direct exposure that would be required.

26. A **grid** is a device composed of uniformly spaced lead foil strips resting on their lateral surface and enclosed in a rigid support framework. It is placed between the patient and the screen-film imaging system when radiographing thicker, denser body parts. The lead foil strips remove scattered radiation from the x-ray beam before it can be photographically effective. The removal of these scattered x-ray photons improves the quality of the radiographic image.

27. A **Bucky mechanism** is a device for moving a grid during an exposure. The grid is suspended in a frame over a tray which holds a cassette during the radiographic exposure. This is done to eliminate the appearance of grid line shadows in the image. The motion of the grid blurs the shadows causing them to become invisible in the image.

28. An **air-gap technique** specifies that the object (part)-film distance be increased thus producing an air-gap between the

object and the film. The increased object-film distance necessitates an increase in source-image distance to prevent magnification of the object in the image. This change necessitates an increase in exposure factors to maintain the radiographic density of the image. This technique is used to reduce the amount of scattered radiation that reaches the image receptor without using a grid. Use of this technique reduces the scattered radiation fog of the image and improves the radiographic image quality without the presence of grid line shadows and about 20% to 25% less radiation dosage than the patient receives if a grid must be used.

29. The **air-gap technique**.

Advantages: Less scattered radiation fog of the image. No grid line shadows in the image. If the radiographic density of the image is maintained, the radiographic contrast of the image is increased, and the visibility of the radiographic detail is enhanced. The patient's radiation dosage is less than if a grid is used to achieve the same image quality.

Disadvantages: Greater x-ray exposure is needed to maintain density if the SID is increased to reduce the magnification resulting from an increased object-image distance. If the SID is not increased, part is magnified significantly in the image; also, patient radiation dosage is greater

107

because the patient is closer to the
radiation source.

30. Exposure technique for an AP projection of the recumbent
abdomen is:

80 mAs	3 mm Al beam filter
80 kVp	100 speed screen-film combination
40" SID	collimation: 14" x 17" field
12:1 Bucky grid	single phase current

a. **Change 100 speed screen to a 200 speed screen:**
The 200 speed screen is two times faster than the 100
speed screen. Same radiographic density in the image
requires the use of 1/2 of the original exposure.

This can be achieve by use of 1/2 of the mAs or by
reducing kVp by 13%. If the kVp is reduced, the kVp used
may not penetrate all of the part adequately; DO NOT
CHANGE kVp!

$$\frac{1}{2}(80 \; mAs) = 40 \; mAs \; should \; be \; used$$

b. **Change 100 speed screen to a 400 speed screen:**
The 400 speed screen is four times faster than the 100
speed screen. Same radiographic density in the image
requires the use of 1/4 of the original exposure.

This can be achieved by use of 1/4 of the mAs or by
reducing the kVp by 13% twice. If the kVp is reduced,

the kVp used may not penetrate all of the part
adequately; DO NOT CHANGE kVp!

$$\frac{1}{4} (80 \; mAs) \; = \; 20 \; mAs \; should \; be \; used$$

c. **Change the 12:1 Bucky grid to an 8:1 Bucky grid.** The
exposure factor for a 12:1 Bucky grid is 5.5; the
exposure factor for an 8:1 Bucky grid is 4.0. The kVp
must be left as it is to ensure penetration of the part.
Change mAs to reduce exposure factors the required
amount.

The ratio of the exposure factors of the grid to be used
to the exposure factor listed originally is 4:5.5. It
is this ratio that determines the new mAs that will be
used to compensate for the lower ratio grid.

$$\frac{4}{5.5} (80 \; mAs) \; = \; \frac{320}{5.5} mAs \; \approx \; 58 \; mAs$$

d. **Change 12:1 Bucky grid to 12:1 stationary grid.** The same
grid ratio is to be used in each case. The only
compensation that must be made is for the change from the
moving to the stationary grid. A moving grid requires
about 15% more exposure than a stationary grid of the
same ratio. This means that the stationary grid should
require about 13% less than the moving grid in this case.

$$80 \; mAs \; - \; 13\% \; (80 \; mAs) \; = \; 80 \; - \; 10.4 \; = \; 69.6 \; mAs$$

Use 69 mAs or 70 mAs to compensate for the change from a moving to a stationary grid.

e. **Change single-phase current to three-phase current.** Change in current generation will require a reduction in exposure to about 1/2 of its initial value.   DO NOT CHANGE kVp!

$$\frac{1}{2}(80 \ mAs) = 40 \ mAs \ should \ be \ used$$

f. **Change 3 mm Al beam filter to 2.5 mm Al beam filter.** There should be very little change in image density with this change so DO NOT CHANGE ANY EXPOSURE FACTORS!

g. **Change 40" SID to 44" SID.**   Exposure factors must be changed to maintain image density. Apply the mathematical calculation for the mAs-distance relationship given in Chapter 11.

$$mAs_2 = \left(\frac{SID_2}{SID_1}\right)^2 \times mAs_1 = \left(\frac{44}{40}\right)^2 \times 80 \ mAs$$

$$= 1.21 \times 80 \ mAs$$

$$= 96.8 \ mAs$$

$$or \ 97 \ mAs \ should \ be \ i$$

31. In any PA projection of a chest film the percent of
    magnification of the heart in the image should be about 8%.
    The exposure technique for a PA projection of a chest which
    measures 28 cm in the AP direction is:

30 mAs	3 mm Al beam filter
90 kVp	100 speed screen
72" SID	single-phase current
8:1 stationary grid	

   a. An **air-gap technique** is requested with an 8" air-gap.
      What is the SID that must be used?

      First, find the original object-image distance. Use
      formulae from Chapter 12.

$$\% \ mag = \frac{OID}{SOD} \times 100\%: \qquad 8\% = \frac{OID}{(72'' - OID)} \times 100\%$$

$$SOD = SID - OID \qquad 0.08 = \frac{x}{(72-x)}$$

$$5.76 - 0.08 \ OID = OID$$

$$1.08 \ OID = 5.76$$

$$OID = \frac{5.76}{1.08} = 5.33''$$

New Case with 8" air-gap:

$$OID = 5.33'' + 8.0'' = 13.33''$$

$$8\% = \frac{13.33}{SID - 13.33} \times 100\%$$

$$0.08 = \frac{13.33}{SID - 13.33}$$

$$0.08 \ SID - 1.0664 = 13.33$$

$$.08 \ SID = 14.3964$$

$$SID = \frac{14.3964}{.08} = 179.955 \ or \ 180'' \ or \ 15'$$

b. What mAs must be used to **compensate for the density loss**
    incurred **by increasing the SID** to the value used in "a"?

$$mAs_2 = \left(\frac{SID_2}{SID_1}\right)^2 \times mAs_1 = \left(\frac{15'}{6'}\right)^2 \times 30 \ mAs$$

$$= 6.25 \times 30 \ mAs$$

$$= 187.5 \ mAs$$

c. **8:1 grid technique is changed to nongrid technique.**
    The exposure factor for an 8:1 grid = 4; exposure
    factor for nongrid = 1. Ratio of exposure factor for
    nongrid to an 8:1 grid is 1:4, or 1/4. Nongrid
    exposure uses 1/4 of mAs used with 8:1 grid.

    mAs_{ng} = 0.25 (187.5 mAs) = 46.875 mAs

d. **Change 100 speed screen to a 400 speed screen.** Use 1/4
    of the mAs found in "C".

    mAs_{400} = 0.25 (46.875 mAs) = 11.72 mAs

e. **Three-phase current used instead of single-phase current.**

This requires a reduction to about one-half of that used with single-phase current.

$$mAs_{3ph} \ = \ 0.5 \ (11.72 \ mAs) \ = \ 5.86 \ mAs$$

f. **Go from 90 kVp to a high kVp technique (>110 kVp)**

      5.86 mAs   nongrid   180" SID   8" air-gap

Use the relationship between mAs and kVp (15% rule) to increase the kVp to a value above 110 kVp.

    5.86 mAs -- x 0.5 ---> 2.93 mAs -- x 0.5 ---> 1.465 mAs

    90   kVp -- + 15% ---> 103.5 kVp -- + 15% --> 119 kVp

g. PA projection of chest measuring 28 cm in the AP direction.

      8" air-gap   1.47 mAs

      nongrid   180" SID

      three-phase current   119 kVp

      400 speed screen

h. Difficulties that may be encountered in a routine radiographic room while trying to accomplish the exposure technique outlined in "g" are:

Primarily, the SID required for this technique, 180" may be impossible to achieve because of the current room size. Most radiography rooms are not that large. All the other factors are likely to be present in most routine radiographic rooms of modern radiography departments or available to them.

i. If the radiographic room is too small to allow the SID needed, the air-gap could be reduced to 6" with very little increase of the radiographic density caused by secondary radiation. The SID that would be required to give 8% magnification of the heart would then be reduced to 153" (12 feet, 9 inches). If the radiologist agrees to accept about 10.5% magnification of the heart shadow in the image, the SID can be further reduced to 120" (10 feet). If the SID is reduced, do not forget the exposure factors must be reduced to maintain the same radiographic density level in the image.

32. a. **Screen speed and the size of the phosphor crystals:** Larger crystals emit more light for a given radiation exposure; therefore the screen is faster. Smaller crystals emit less light and produce slower screens.

   b. **Screen speed and the thickness of the phosphor crystal layers:** Thicker layers of phosphor crystals emit more light per given radiation exposure and these screens are faster. Thinner layers of crystals emit less light and produce slower speed screens.

   c. **Screen speed and the addition of coloring dye** to the binder material suspending and holding the phosphor crystals: Coloring dye in the binder material hinders the light rays from the deeper parts of the phosphor crystal layer in their efforts to emerge from the screen. This addition to the binder material slows the screen speed.

   d. **Screen speed and the use of a reflective layer in intensifying screens:** The reflective layer redirects light photons emitted in its direction back toward the

film. The presence of a reflective layer in an
intensifying screen increases the speed of that screen.

e. **Screen speed and the kV level used for radiographic
    exposures:** In calcium tungstate screens the speed
    undergoes changes with the various kV levels used for an
    exposure. The screen speed is slower below 70 kVp to 75
    kVp. At the 70 kVp to 80 kVp range it becomes relatively
    constant, but any increase in kVp does continue to elicit
    some increase in screen response. A rare earth phosphor
    screen demonstrates maximum speed at about 80 kVp. At
    lower and higher levels of kV the screen exhibits less
    speed.

f. **Screen speed and the types of phosphor crystals used** in
    the intensifying screen: Calcium tungstate crystals
    absorb about 20% of the incident x-ray photon energy and
    convert about 5% of this to light. Hypothetically, if
    there are 100 x-ray photons in the incident beam, 20 of
    them are absorbed and only 1 is actually converted to
    light to expose the film.

Rare earth phosphor crystals absorb about 60% of the
incident x-ray photon energy and convert about 20% of
this to light. In the same hypothetical situation with
100 incident x-ray photons and using these phosphors, 60
would be absorbed and 12 of these would be converted to
light and expose the film.

Rare earth screens exhibit a greater screen speed than

calcium tungstate screens.

33. The **photostimulable phosphor screen** is the one used in computed radiographic imaging.

34. The photostimulable screen is flooded with light which erases any image remaining from a previous exposure. When exposed to x-rays, all electrons in the phosphor are excited (raised to a higher energy state). About half will return immediately to the original energy state. The others are trapped and form the basis for the latent image. The screen must be put into a special reader to retrieve a visible image. This reader uses a laser light to scan the screen. The trapped electrons absorb the laser light energy thus freeing themselves. As the electron frees itself (returns to a lower energy level) it emits a light photon. The light emitted is transmitted to a remote photomultiplier tube where a continuous point-by-point scan of the image is the output result. The output is an electrical signal corresponding to the x-rays absorbed by the screen while being exposed to the radiation that passed through the part. The signal is amplified, converted to a digital signal, and stored in a computer. The computer can take the digital signal and reconvert it to an analog image that can be viewed by various conventional means.

This development appears to be able to require fewer film in order to visualize the part. It means there will be less need for repeat radiographic exposures because of poor choice of exposure factors. The computer can, within some limits, alter the image quality without repeating the exposure. This provides a wider range of radiation exposures which can be used to obtain good quality images. This indicates that the radiation dosage to the general public will be reduced and the radiography department can operate more economically and efficiently.

35. A lateral cervical spine at an SID of 72" should not require the use of a grid exposure technique. The part radiographed is, because of its position relative to the film surface, removed from the image receptor surface by about 8" to 10". This is, in effect, an air-gap technique and much of the secondary radiation produced does not strike the film to produce scattered radiation fog. Most of the scattered radiation is eliminated without the increase in exposure to the patient that would be required with the use of a grid.

CHAPTER 14 SOLUTIONS

1. Higher atomic number materials attenuate or absorb a greater percentage of the beam than lower atomic number materials.

2. The thicker the body part the greater the attenuation of the beam.

3. Muscle has a higher atomic number and a greater tissue density than fat. As a result, muscle attenuates the beam more than fat. Radiographic density will decrease with muscle because it absorbs more photons than fat.

4. The body is composed of approximately 62% muscle, 15% fat and 23% bone. Approximately 40% of the total body weight is composed of muscle by age 17.

5.	By being familiar with pathological conditions the radiographer will be able to more effectively evaluate when and how the exposure factors are adjusted in order to obtain the best possible image.

6.	Additive pathology results from production of bone making the part harder to penetrate; as a result, an increase in exposure factor is required because a greater attenuation of the beam occurs.

Destructive pathology results from loss of bone making it easier to penetrate. This condition requires a decrease in exposure factors because less attenuation of the beam occurs.

7.	Because each individual is different and no two people are identical. By having an accurate clinical history available, the radiographer can use this information along with their clinical expertise to do whatever is necessary (adjust exposure factors and/or positioning techniques) to obtain a diagnostic image in order for the radiologist to make a proper diagnosis.

8.	a.	**Paget's disease** - requires an increase in exposure factors to compensate for production of bone.

	b.	**Bowel obstruction** - requires a decrease in exposure factors to compensate for excessive gas present in the abdominal cavity.

	c.	**Ascites** - requires an increase in exposure factors as a result of fluid in the peritoneal cavity. Radiographer should note that a high ratio grid may be necessary to maintain high film quality as a result of production of scatter radiation when kVp is increased to improve penetration.

   d. **Emphysema** - requires a decrease in exposure factors as result of excess air in the thoracic cavity. Radiographer should note that the extent of the disease and not is its presence determines how much exposure factors are adjusted.

9.   In general when performing bone radiography, a short scale-high contrast is desired. This can be accomplished by the use of a low kVp technique.

10. a. **Sthenic habitus** is the average body build that comprises approximately 50% of the population.

   b. **Hyposthenic habitus** - modification of the asthenic type, it is more toward the sthenic type but slender build. Approximately 35% of individuals are of this body build.

   c. **Asthenic habitus** - extremely slender build with emaciated body tissue. This type of individual represents approximately 10% of the population.

   d. **Hypersthenic habitus** - massive or heavy body build. 5% of persons fall into this category.

CHAPTER 15 SOLUTIONS

   1. c

   2. b

   3. a

   4. b

   5. d

   6. b

7. a

8. d

9. a

10. c

EXERCISE SOLUTIONS

1. (a) 25,   (b) 100,   (c) 144

2. (a) 750,   (b) 5,000, (c) 7200

3. Input phosphor

   Photocathode

   Electrostatic lens

   Anode

   Output screen

4. Image brightness is usually controlled through the use of mAs
   and kVp. In older equipment, this may be operator-
   controlled; in newer equipment a photocell sets the mAs and
   kVp. Also the video signal or vidicon plate may be adjusted
   to compensate for image brightness.

5. Factors affecting the resolution of the image are the video
   monitor, minification gain, electrostatic focal spot, the
   diameter of the input and output screen, OID, and phosphor
   size and thickness. TV monitors can resolve only 1-2 lp/mm,
   and are thus both the primary factor and the weakest link in
   the imaging chain.

6. The interlace method uses the first field to scan even
   numbered lines. A second field scans odd numbered lines.
   This produces a new image every 1/60 second. Thus, the
   first scan scans alternating 262 1/2 lines in the first 1/60

second, the second scan the next alternating 262 1/2 lines. This removes flicker from the image.

7. The main disadavantages of mirror systems are loss of light (limiting the effectiveness of the image intensifier) and only one viewer can observe the image at any one time. Advantages that the monitor possesses over the mirror viewing system include many viewers possible, a lower patient dose, and increased brightness. Monitors are more expensive and require more space.

8. Spot films offer the best quality but have a relatively high patient dose using radiographic sheet film and processors with the slowest framing frequencies. Photospot cameras have good quality, a low patient dose using radiographic film and processors, and a framing frequency faster than spot films. Cine also has good quality, uses roll film with a low patient dose, and requires a special processor. It provides a faster framing frequency than the first two, which is used to make movies of moving organs such as the heart. Videotape and disk have the poorest quality and a low patient dose. They require no processor, with tape being reusable.

9. Quantum mottle is a grainy or blotchy appearance caused by insufficient radiation to produce a uniform image. Since x-rays are emitted at random, variations in x-ray intensity are most at low mAs values. Mottle is a problem in fluoroscopy as units operate based on the minimum number of photons to activate the fluoroscopic screen through ABS.

10. With multifield image intensifiers capable of operating in several modes, the smaller the mode used, the less the

minification. In a dual-field intensifier capable of 6" and 9" mode, the voltage is increased in the 6" mode, focusing the electrons farther away from the output phosphor. In this mode, the optical system can only see the central part of the image derived from the central 6" of the input phosphor. This image is less minified and therefore appears to be magnified on the monitor. Thus, smaller modes provide a larger image; however, exposure factors and patient dose must be increased to compensate for the loss in brightness.

CHAPTER 16 SOLUTIONS

1. Remove any patient and notify the supervisor.
2. a. The tube crane is *not* in the detent for the automatic collimator.
   b. The Bucky tray is *not* making contact with the automatic collimator detector plug.
3. The image was produced using a cassette in the inverted or "up-side-down" position. The wrinkles are small cracks or flexes in the lead foil.
4. Excessively low kVp.
5. Clear letters on a dark background.
6. The image is light because the activated cell is *not* under the bony anatomy of interest.
7. The image will be light and will exhibit vertical lines or streaks caused by the cutoff.
8. The serviceman did not replace the added filter. The beam is underfiltered, and the beam intensity is high.
9. The image will be dark. The smaller beam will produce less

scatter. The AEC detector will be exposed to less radiation and will drive the timer longer.

10. Turn off the power at the wall switch or circuit breaker, and notify the supervisor.

CHAPTER 17 SOLUTIONS

1. Quality assurance and quality control are structured measures to monitor and control the many variables that influence the quality of radiographic images.

2. Quality control is one aspect of total quality assurance. Quality control usually refers to technical tests used to monitor the performance of equipment.

3. The four major components of processor quality control are: (1) chemical activity, ensured by accurate mixing of the chemical solutions and routine checking of replenishment rates and chemical activity; (2) cleaning; (3) maintenance; and (4) monitoring, in three steps that require a daily routine.

4. The following values are taken:
   "S" is the speed index step, which should have a density near 1.2, (1.0 above base plus fog).
   "H" is a high density step, which should have a density near 2.2 (2.0 above base plus fog).
   "L" is a low density step, which should have a density near 45 (0.25 above base plus fog).
   "H" minus "L" is the contrast index. The base plus fog is measured in the clear area adjacent to the strip.

5. The level and number of quality control tests performed is

dependent on the facility and the training of technical personnel. A small clinic may perform only very basic first- and second-level tests. A large hospital will have a comprehensive program that includes all levels of tests. Routine tests include daily penetrometer (step wedge) checks; processor quality control, to include chemical activity, cleaning and maintenance, and monitoring; mAs reciprocity using a step-wedge x-ray beam/light beam congruence; x-ray beam and Bucky tray alignment; and routine physical or visual evaluations.

6. a. The 8 cent test is performed for congruence of the light beam and x-ray beam.

    b. mAs reciprocity determines whether combinations of mA and time that produce the same mAs produce the same exposure holding all other variables equal.

    c. The star pattern provides information about the size of the focal spot.

    d. The wire mesh test determines screen/film contact.

7. The goals of quality assurance and quality control are (1) to reduce patient dose, (2) to minimize the cost of examinations, and (3), to increase the quality of patient care.

8. Third-level test involving disassembly are not normally performed by technologists unless they have secured advanced training.

9. Determination of the half value layer (HVL) may be used as a reference standard for kVp calibration or tube aging evidenced by hardening of the beam as a result of tungsten

deposits on the inside of the glass tube housing.

10. Single-phase.

CHAPTER 18 SOLUTIONS

1. B, B, A, B, A

2. T, F, F, T

3. b

4. b

5. a

6. d

7. c

8. c

9. a

10. b

11. c

12. c

13. c

14. a

15. d

EXERCISE SOLUTIONS

1. In general, as LET increases, so does RBE. Thus high LET radiations such as alpha and beta also have a high RBE. Low LET radiations such as x-ray and gamma have a low RBE.

2. 1/2 or 0.5. This means that the test radiation is half as effective as the 250 keV x-ray.

3. Hematologic cells are constantly being produced, with life

spans that vary from a few days to about 4 months. Lymphocytes are considered to be one of the two most sensitive cells in the body to radiation, whereas erythrocytes, with a relatively long life span and a fairly high degree of differentiation, are among the least radiosensitive cells in the body. Their stem cells, erythroblasts, on the other hand, are more radiosensitive.

4. Effects such as cellular carcinogenesis, tissue-level effects, host effects, and clinical cancer induction are poorly understood because of confounding and synergistic effects that may not be due to radiation. They could be due to exposure to other diseases or risk agents such as chemicals or smoking.

5. Muller's studies indicated that: (1) there was no increase in the quality of mutations or the types of observed mutations; (2) most mutations observed were recessive; (3) no threshold was observed; and (4) that mutations were single-hit phenomena and were cumulative in nature.

The "megamouse" experiments differed manily in that a dose-rate effect was seen; a given dose extended over a long period of time showed less effects genetically than one large dose.

6. The GSD assumes that the long-term effects of radiation can be averaged over a population. It is calculated by a formula that looks at the average gonadal dose per examination, the number of persons receiving x-ray examinations, the total number of persons in the population, and the expected number

of future children per person. It is an average calculated from actual gonadal doses received by the whole population.

7. The principle effects of radiation on an embryo or fetus are: (1) embryonic, fetal, or neonatal death; (2) malformations; (3) retardation of growth; (4) congenital defects; and (5) cancer induction. Two factors influence the effects of radiation on the embryo and fetus: the stage of development and the radiation dose.

8. Since the central nervous system (CNS) remains highly undifferentiated in the fetus, large doses of radiation can have a variety of effects on the CNS. Radiosensitivity begins to decrease at 20 weeks, but the fetus then becomes more susceptible to late effects and CNS effects.

9. Diminished growth and development is theoretically possible at all stages but primarily will occur during the latter part of gestation and possibly during the very early stages of gestation. Growth retardation will not be seen in the preimplantation stage, will be temporary with irradiation in the organogenesis stage, and permanent if the fetus is irradiated during the fetal stage. During the later stages this is thought to be due to cell depletion with a consequent reduction in size. No congenital abnormalities are observed, but the individual will have a somewhat reduced physical size.

10. Point mutations (also known as a gene mutation) are not microscopically detectable but may result in an altered phenotype. This results from the substitution of a single amino acid in its protein structure, which may arise from a

single alteration along the sequence of DNA bases.

Radiations may cause strand breakage of DNA, which in turn, if not returned to the exact original sequence of bases, would cause a mutation of the broken section of the DNA. Point mutations may give rise to a nonsense codon or a missense codon, which would provide no useful information for that particular segment of DNA.

Frameshift mutations result from the gain or loss of one or more DNA bases. This may alter the interpretation of an extended length of the DNA sequence and, therefore, provide a greater probability for the induction of a detectable change.

CHAPTER 19 SOLUTIONS

1. a
2. a
3. b
4. a
5. d
6. b
7. d
8. a
9. a
10. c

EXERCISE SOLUTIONS

1. The primary difference between the two types of curves is that the linear, non-threshold curve shows a proportional increase in effects with a proportional increase in dose. It also assumed that any dose of radiation can have an effect. A non-linear curve does not show a proportional increase in effects with dose and has a threshold, a dose below which no effects occur.

2. Stochastic effects show an increase in effects in proportion to radiation dose of the entire population. They do not exhibit a threshold and are associated with the linear and the linear-quadratic dose-response curves. Radiation risks from diagnostic imaging, with the exception of in utero exposure of a viable fetus, are considered to be stochastic as well as heredity effects and carcinogenesis.

   Nonstochastic effects increase in severity with dose, and there is a threshold assumed. It is also sometimes called the certainty effect and is associated with high doses. Cataract induction, nonmalignant damage to skin, hematologic deficiences, and impairment to fertility are considered nonstochastic effects.

3. Early radiation protection principles were based on the experiences of early radiation workers and patients. Effects observed were used to formulate guidelines for radiation protection.

4. The 10-25 rule uses common sense and principles of radiobiology to determine what should be done following

radiation exposure in utero. Under this rule, less than 10 rad should never be an indication to terminate a pregnancy. Between 10 and 25 rad is a "gray area" in which the determination to terminate a pregnancy will depend on the time of exposure. Above 25 rad termination of a pregnancy should be considered.

5. The primary study used to determine the potential effects of radiation on the breast comes from exposures to survivors of the atomic bomb. Since it is not a direct comparison (e.g., mammography was not studied), there is a degree of uncertainty associated with the study.

6. There are few detriments associated with radiography. As noted earlier in the chapter, radiation exposure at 500 mrem per year from age 20 is only associated with 7 days of life expectancy lost. This is much safer than occupations such as coal mining or construction work.

The potential benefits associated with radiography can be great, although this of course depends on the individual. The potential to help others is the main reason why individuals enter this profession. The small risk must be balanced with the potential to do great good for the health of the population.

7 This study lacked, first, a control group with which to compare normal cancer incidence. Second, the study had not been conducted over a long enough time to determine longitudinal effects.

CHAPTER 20 SOLUTIONS

1. a. the International Commission on Radiological Protection (ICRP)

   b. the National Council on Radiation Protection and Measurements (NCRP)

   c. the U.S. Nuclear Regulatory Commission (NRC) and individual State Health Departments

2. Absorbed Dose = (Exposure)(appropriate f-Factor)

   then

   Dose Equivalent = (Absorbed Dose)(appropriate

   quality Factor)

3. a. Absorbed Dose = Exposure x (f-Factor)

   $$= (60 \text{ R})(0.95)$$

   $$= 57 \text{ rad}$$

   b. Dose Equivalent = Absorbed Dose x Quality Factor

   $$= (57 \text{ rads})(1)$$

   $$= 57 \text{ rem}$$

   c. Since the maximum effective dose equivalent to the hands should not exceed 50 rem, this limit has been exceeded.

4. a. Absorbed Dose = Exposure x (f-Factor)

   $$= (9 \times 10^{-4} \text{ coulomb/kg})(37)$$

   $$= 3.33 \times 10^{-2} \text{ Gy}$$

   $$= 33.3 \text{ mGy}$$

   b. Dose Equivalent = Absorbed Dose x Quality Factor

   $$= (33.3 \text{ mGy})(1)$$

   $$= 33.3 \text{ mSv}$$

c. Since the maximum effective dose equivalent to the whole body is set at 50 mSv, this limit has not been exceeded by this exposure.

5. a. $10^2 \, mSv \times \dfrac{1 \, Sv}{10^3 \, mSv} \times \dfrac{10^2 \, rem}{Sv} = 10 \, rem$

b. $2 \, mrem \times \dfrac{1 \, rem}{10^3 \, mrem} \times \dfrac{1 \, Sv}{10^2 \, rem} \times \dfrac{10^3 \, mSv}{1 \, Sv} = 0.02 \, mSv$

c. $10 \, cGy \times \dfrac{1 \, Gy}{10^2 \, cGy} \times \dfrac{10^2 \, rad}{1 \, Gy} = 10 \, rad$

d. $400 \, mrem \times \dfrac{1 \, rem}{10^3 \, mrem} \times \dfrac{1 \, Sv}{10^2 \, rem} \times \dfrac{10^3 \, mSv}{1 \, Sv} = 4 \, mSv$

e $600 \, R \times \dfrac{\dfrac{1 \, coul}{kg}}{3876 \, R} \approx 0.155 \dfrac{coul}{kg}$

6. ALARA refers to the basic philosophy of radiation protection of taking appropriate action to keep one's occupational radiation exposure as low as reasonably achievable.

7. Occupational radiation exposure is measured using personnel dosimetry devices such as film badges, TLDs, or pocket dosimeters.

8. Occupational exposure can be easily determined from the printed dosimetry report which should be posted in the department each month.

9. **Film badges** - occupational exposure is determined by the degree of darkening of the film when it is processed; the darker the film the more exposure the wearer has received.

TLDs - utilizes a crystal (LiF or CaF$_2$) which absorbs radiation energy entering the crystal; when the crystal is heated (or annealed), light is given off in proportion to the energy absorbed

Pocket dosimeters - work on the principle of the electroscope; when fully charged using a charging base, a charged fiber moves to zero position on scale; as radiation enters and produces ion pairs within the device, charge is neutralized in proportion to total dose received; cumulative exposure is read directly off the scale

10. No. Personal medical or dental x-rays do not constitute occupational radiation exposure.

11. See Table 20-4 for a listing of advantages and disadvantages of each type dosimetry device

12. For a monthly occupational limit for the whole body, divide the allowable annual limits by 12:

$$monthly\ occupational\ limit = \frac{5000\ mrem}{12} \approx 416.6\ mrem$$

$$or\ \frac{50\ mSv}{12} \approx 4.16\ mSv$$

13. Time, distance, and use of appropriate shielding.

14. a. Grave Danger: Very High Radiation Area

    b. Caution: Radiation Area

    c. Caution: Radioactive Materials

    d. DOT Class II Label

    e. DOT Class III Label

    f. Caution: Radiation Area

15. a. A primary barrier is used to attenuate radiation from the primary beam of an x-ray unit.

    A secondary barrier is designed to attenuate leakage and secondary radiation from an x-ray unit.

    b. Primary barriers are determined by which particular walls of an imaging room will have the x-ray unit directed toward them. All other walls are considered to be secondary barriers.

    c. Primary barriers are thicker or have more shielding materials in them compared with secondary barriers.

16. In order to minimize fetal radiation exposure

    a. The technologist may not wish to participate in fluoroscopic procedures.

    b. The technologist may choose to wear a lead apron when working with radiation sources.

    c. The technologist may wish to wear 2 film badges--one at collar level, one at waist level (under the Pb apron to monitor fetal exposure).

EXERCISE SOLUTIONS

1.
$$I_1 d_1^2 = I_2 d_2^2$$

$$\left(50\frac{mR}{hr}\right)(3m)^2 = \left(2\frac{mR}{hr}\right)(d_2^2)$$

$$d_2^2 = \left(\frac{50\frac{mR}{hr}}{2\frac{mR}{hr}}\right)(3m)^2$$

$$d_2^2 = (25)(9m^2) = 225\ m^2$$

$$d_2 = 15\ m$$

2. Dose Rate $= \dfrac{Dose}{Time}$

   therefore, time $= \dfrac{Dose}{Dose\ rate}$

   $$= \frac{25mrem}{20\frac{mrem}{hr}}$$

   $$= 0.8\ hr \quad or \quad 48\ minutes$$

   Note: For photons, we make the approximation that roentgens $\approx$ rad = rem

3. a. Dose equivalent = (10 rad)(20)

   $\qquad\qquad\qquad = 200$ rem

   b. Dose equivalent = (3 rad)(5)

   $\qquad\qquad\qquad = 15$ rem

   c. Dose equivalent = (5 cGy)(1)

   $\qquad\qquad\qquad = 5$ cSv

   d. Absorbed dose $= (15\ R)(1) = 15$ rad;

   then, dose equivalent = (15 rad)(1) = 15 rem

135

e.   Absorbed dose = (3.5 R)(1) = 3.5 rad

then dose equivalent = (3.5 rad)(1) = 3.5 rem

4. a.

$$I = I_o(0.5)^N$$

$$= \left(120\,\frac{mR}{hr}\right)(0.5)^{\frac{1\ mm}{0.24\ mm}}$$

$$= \left(120\,\frac{mR}{hr}\right)(0.5)^{4.17}$$

$$= \left(120\,\frac{mR}{hr}\right)(0.056)$$

$$\approx 6.7\,\frac{mR}{hr}$$

b.

$$I = I_o(0.5)^N$$

$$\frac{I}{I_o} = (0.5)^N$$

$$\frac{2}{120} = (0.5)^N$$

$$0.017 = (0.5)^N$$

$$\ln(0.017) = N\,\ln(0.5)$$

$$-4.075 \approx N(-0.693)$$

$$N = \frac{-4.075}{-0.693} \approx 5.88\ HVLs\ needed$$

thickness needed = (5.88)(1.5 mm concrete)

≈ 8.82 mm of concrete

c.

$$\frac{I}{I_o} = (0.5)^N$$

$$0.01 = (0.5)^N$$

$$\ln(0.01) = N\,\ln(0.5)$$

$$-4.605 = N(-0.693)$$

$$N = \frac{-4.605}{-0.693} \approx 6.65\ HVLs$$

5. a.

$$N = \frac{0.25 \ mm}{0.19 \frac{mm}{HVL}} \approx 1.32 \ HVLs$$

$$\frac{I}{I_o} = (0.5)^{1.32} \approx 0.4005$$

Thus 40% of the incident radiation is transmitted.

b.

$$N = \frac{0.50 \ mm}{0.19 \frac{mm}{HVL}} \approx 2.63 HVLs$$

$$\frac{I}{I_o} = (0.5)^{2.63} \approx 0.1615$$

Thus 16% of the incident radiation is transmitted.

c.

$$N = \frac{1.00 \ mm}{0.19 \frac{mm}{HVL}} \approx 5.26 HVLs$$

$$\frac{I}{I_o} = (0.5)^{5.26} \approx 0.026$$

Thus ~2.6% of the incident radiation is transmitted.

CHAPTER 21 SOLUTIONS

1. a

2. d

3. d

4. d

5. a

6. c

7. a

8. c

9. a

10. c

EXERCISE SOLUTIONS

1. Step 1: mAs is being halved; therefore, the intensity
    due to mAs will <u>decrease</u> to one-half original
    value.

$$\frac{mAs_1}{mAs_2} = \frac{I_1}{I_2}$$

$$\frac{10}{5} = \frac{55}{x}$$

$$x = 27.5 \; mR$$

Step 2: kVp is being increased. Thus intensity will
now *increase* as follows:

$$\left(\frac{70}{80}\right)^2 = \frac{27.5}{x}$$

x = 31.4 mR, a total decrease of 23.6 mR

2. The more effective change would be stepping back to 2 meters
as this would cut radiation intensity by one-fourth to 5
mrad. Adding a half-value layer apron would only cut dose in
half to 10 mrad. The best answer might be to do both, which
would cut dose by one-eighth to 2.5 mrad.

3. There is no one answer to this question. The following
should be looked for:

a. The policy should contain a section stating the previous exposure history of the radiographer (e.g., I, the undersigned, realize that my previous exposure has been _____).

b. The radiographer should be provided with the option of wearing an additional monitor.

c. A section should indicate the responsibilities of the radiographer to practice safely and of the employer to provide a safe environment.

d. The NCRP recommended limit of 0.5 should be listed as a guide.

e. The overall tone of the document should indicate that decisions (such as rotation out of fluoroscopy and mobile radiography) are to be made jointly between the employer and worker.

4. Selection of kilovoltage is the most effective method of limiting patient dose of those items easily selectable by the radiographer. This is illustrated in question 1, above.

   The second most effective technique for reducing patient dose is the use of faster film/screen combinations. Doubling screen speed will effectively limit patient dose (cut it in half), but this technique is not as often under the control of the radiographer.

5. The ultimate goal of state licensing and voluntary certification is protection of the patient. By providing patients with competent practitioners who understand and are able to practice safe radiation protection, the health of the population is protected.

6. By establishing communication, it is easier to secure patient consent. If patients understand the reason behind procedures and are involved in the examination, they will cooperate.

7. The factors that will influence repeat rate include the experience level of the radiographer and the radiologist's view of image quality. Also a departmental quality assurance program is designed to minimize repeats, which results in higher image quality and patient protection.

8. Any adult (unless they have had their civil rights removed) can refuse an examination. The radiographer should never advocate refusal to a patient but should instead gently try to emphasize the concept of safe radiation protection and risk being counterbalanced by the benefit of radiography.

9. Mobile radiography takes a radiation hazard into a place not set up for radiation protection. Often family, other patients, and nurses must be educated in proper radiation protection. Contact in the patient unit often gives the radiographer the opportunity to take advantage of that brief moment to teach safe radiation protection and the professional role of the radiographer in radiation protection.

10. The balance between mA and time is extremely important in phototiming (using automatic exposure controls). To minimize the possibility of grossly overexposing the patient. Some authorities recommend using only 1.5 times the expected mAs. Also, phototiming is not always as precisely reproducible as manual timing. Positioning must

be duplicated exactly for the repeat exposure.

CHAPTER 22 SOLUTIONS

1. CT images, unlike conventional radiography, are not formed by the interaction of transmitted x-rays with radiographic film. Instead transmission data is acquired at various angles, stored within the computer, and then used to reconstruct the final image. The data can be mathematically manipulated to produce additional images in other body planes. Image contrast can also be electronically adjusted without making additional exposures.

2. Nuclear medicine images are used to evaluate organ function. This is referred to as physiological imaging.

3. Diagnostic radiography typically utilizes x-rays in the energy range of ~60 keV - 100 keV. ^{99m}Tc emits gamma photons of 140 keV. The energies used by both modalities are comparable.

4. In addition to standard radiation protection practices, the nuclear medicine technologist must also be concerned with radioactive contamination--the spread of radioactive materials to places where it should not be.

5. The radiation used in MRI falls into the radiofrequency (RF) portion of the electromagnetic energy spectrum. RF radiation is nonionizing and much lower in energy ($~10^{-6}$eV - 10^{-8}eV) than conventional x-rays used for medical imaging.

6. MRI holds several advantages: (1) MRI does not use ionizing radiation; (2) MRI is the only imaging modality which can obtain images in almost any body plane without the

need to reposition the patient; (3) MRI has the potential to visualize chemical changes within the body which possibly could indicate the presence of pathology; (4) Bone is invisible on proton (hydrogen) MR images; (5) Fluid filled structures (e.g., cysts) can be detected using proton density imaging techniques.

7. Exposure to radiofrequency radiation and strong magnetic fields are still points of concern for potential long-range biological effects.

8. Infrared (Heat) radiation.

9. Thermography does not utilize ionizing radiation and is a noninvasive imaging technique.

Worksheet 2-1: Fractions, Decimals, Ratios, and Proportions

I. Fractions

1. $\dfrac{9}{5}$

2. $\dfrac{2}{3}+\dfrac{3}{6}+\dfrac{1}{12} = \dfrac{8}{12}+\dfrac{6}{12}+\dfrac{1}{12} = \dfrac{15}{12}$

3. $\dfrac{1}{2}+\dfrac{2}{3}+\dfrac{3}{4} = \dfrac{6}{12}+\dfrac{8}{12}+\dfrac{9}{12} = \dfrac{23}{12}$

4. $\dfrac{4}{5} \div \dfrac{3}{5} = \dfrac{4}{5} \times \dfrac{5}{3} = \dfrac{4}{3}$

5. $\dfrac{4}{9} \div \dfrac{7}{16} = \dfrac{4}{9} \times \dfrac{16}{7} = \dfrac{64}{63}$

6. $\dfrac{8}{9} \div \dfrac{3}{5} = \dfrac{8}{9} \times \dfrac{5}{3} = \dfrac{40}{27}$

II. Decimals

1.a. $\dfrac{5}{10} = 0.5$

b. $\dfrac{8}{100} = 0.08$

c. $\dfrac{6}{10,000} = 0.0006$

d. $\dfrac{8}{125} = 0.064$ (*obtain with calculator*)

2.a. $0.01 = \dfrac{1}{100}$

143

b. $0.250 = \dfrac{250}{1000} = \dfrac{25}{100} = \dfrac{1}{4}$

c.

$0.125 = \dfrac{125}{1000} = \dfrac{1}{8}$

d. $0.0005 = \dfrac{5}{10,000} = \dfrac{1}{2000}$

III. Alegebraic Relations

1.

$$x+4-7 = -10+4-x$$

$$x-3 = -6-x$$

$$x+x = -6+3$$

$$2x = -3$$

$$x = -\dfrac{3}{2}$$

2.

$$\dfrac{x}{3} = \dfrac{7}{9}$$

$$9 \cdot x = 3 \cdot 7$$

$$9x = 21$$

$$x = \dfrac{21}{9} = \dfrac{7}{3}$$

3.

$$\dfrac{4}{x} = \dfrac{6+2}{8}$$

$$\dfrac{4}{x} = \dfrac{8}{8}$$

$$\dfrac{4}{x} = 1$$

$$4 = x \cdot 1$$

$$x = 4$$

4.

$$\frac{x+3}{5} = -10 + \frac{5}{3}$$

$$\frac{x+3}{5} = -\frac{30}{3} + \frac{5}{3}$$

$$\frac{x+3}{5} = -\frac{25}{3}$$

$$3(x+3) = -25(5)$$

$$3x+9 = -125$$

$$3x = -125-9 = -134$$

$$x = -\frac{134}{3}$$

5.

$$\frac{1}{x} = \frac{1}{5} + \frac{1}{20}$$

$$\frac{1}{x} = \frac{4}{20} + \frac{1}{20}$$

$$\frac{1}{x} = \frac{5}{20}$$

$$x = \frac{20}{5} = 4$$

6.

$$\frac{1}{10} = \frac{1}{x} + \frac{1}{20}$$

$$\frac{1}{10} - \frac{1}{20} = \frac{1}{x}$$

$$\frac{2}{20} - \frac{1}{20} = \frac{1}{x}$$

$$\frac{1}{20} = \frac{1}{x}$$

$$x = \frac{20}{1} = 20$$

IV.   Ratios and Proportions

1.
$$\frac{x}{7} = \frac{3}{4}$$

$$4 \cdot x = 3 \cdot 7$$

$$4x = 21$$

$$X = \frac{21}{4}$$

2.
$$\frac{4}{9} = \frac{3}{x}$$

$$4 \cdot x = 3 \cdot 9$$

$$4x = 27$$

$$x = \frac{27}{4}$$

3.
$$\frac{5}{7} = \frac{x}{2}$$

$$7 \cdot x = 5 \cdot 2$$

$$7x = 10$$

$$x = \frac{10}{7}$$

4.
$$\frac{x+2}{3} = \frac{5}{8}$$

$$8(x+2) = 5 \cdot 3$$

$$8x + 16 = 15$$

$$8x = 15 - 16 = -1$$

$$x = -\frac{1}{8}$$

Worksheet 2-2:   Scientific Notation

I.   1. 8.3×10^{-4}

2. 1.008×10^{6}

3. 1×10^{0}

4. 1.087×10^4

5. 5.2×10^{-7}

II.   1. 1.2×10^9

2. 3×10^6

3. 9×10^{10}

4. 1.2×10^{-9}

5. 1.2×10^9

6. 4×10^{-8}

7. 5×10^2

8. 6.4×10^{-5}

9. 5×10^5

10. 1.5×10^1

Worksheet 2-3:   Algebraic Equations

1.
$$5x + 10 = 135$$
$$5x = 135 - 10 = 125$$
$$x = \frac{125}{5} = 25$$

2.
$$80x = 400$$
$$x = \frac{400}{80} = 5$$

3.
$$\frac{1}{2}x + 8 = 20+5$$
$$\frac{1}{2}x = 25-8 = 17$$
$$x = 2(17) = 34$$

4.
$$\frac{3}{4}x = 24$$
$$x = \left(\frac{4}{3}\right)(24) = 32$$

5.

$$\frac{1}{x} = \frac{1}{5} + \frac{1}{2}$$

$$\frac{1}{x} = \frac{2}{10} + \frac{5}{10} = \frac{7}{10}$$

$$\frac{x}{1} = \frac{10}{7}$$

$$x = \frac{10}{7}$$

6.

$$\frac{3}{4} = \frac{2}{x} + \frac{1}{2}$$

$$\frac{2}{x} = \frac{3}{4} - \frac{1}{2}$$

$$\frac{2}{x} = \frac{3}{4} - \frac{2}{4} = \frac{1}{4}$$

$$\frac{2}{x} = \frac{1}{4}$$

$$\frac{x}{2} = \frac{4}{1}$$

$$x = 2(4) = 8$$

7.

$$x^2 = 45$$

$$x = \sqrt{45} \approx 6.7$$

8.

$$8x^2 = 64$$

$$x^2 = \frac{64}{8} = 8$$

$$x = \sqrt{8} \approx 2.8$$

9.

$$2x^2 - 10 = 25$$

$$2x^2 = 25 + 10 = 35$$

$$x^2 = \frac{35}{2} = 17.5$$

$$x = \sqrt{17.5} \approx 4.2$$

10.

$$2(3x)^2 = 36$$

$$(3x)^2 = \frac{36}{2} = 18$$

$$3x = \sqrt{18} \approx 4.2$$

$$x \approx \frac{1}{3}(4.2) \approx 1.4$$

Worksheet 2-4: Logarithmic and Exponential Equations

I.   Logs

   1.   1

   2.   3

   3.   4

   4.   1.934

   5.   3.199

   6.   1

   7.   4.454

   8.   7.365

   9.   4.605

  10.   9.21

II.   Exponents

   1.   100,000

   2.   100

   3.   316.2

   4.   1000

   5.   6309.6

   6.   0.25

   7.   4

   8.   0.177

   9.   7.388

10. 40.43

III. Logarithmic Equations

1.
$$\log_{10} x = 3.7$$
$$\Rightarrow 10^{3.7} = x$$
$$x = 5011.9$$

2.
$$4 \log x = 20$$
$$\log x = \frac{1}{4}(20) = 5$$
$$\Rightarrow 10^5 = x$$

3.
$$\frac{1}{10} \ln x = -0.04$$
$$\ln_e x = (10)(-0.04) = -0.4$$
$$\Rightarrow e^{-0.4} = x$$
$$x = (2.718)^{-0.4} = 0.67$$

4.
$$2 \ln 25 = x$$
$$2(3.219) \approx x$$
$$x \approx 6.438$$

5.
$$x = \frac{1}{4} \ln 20$$
$$= \frac{1}{4}(2.996)$$
$$\approx 0.749$$

IV. Exponential Equations

1.
$$27 = 4e^x$$
$$e^x = \frac{1}{4}(27) = 6.75$$

To solve, take the natural log (i.e., ln) of both sides:

$$\ln(e^x) = \ln 6.75$$

$$\Rightarrow x \ln e = \ln 6.75$$

$$x(1) \approx 1.91$$

$$x \approx 1.91$$

2.

$$10 = e^{-x}$$

Take ln *of both sides*:

$$\ln 10 = \ln(e^{-x})$$

$$\ln 10 = (-x)\ln e$$

$$2.3 = -x(1)$$

$$x = -2.3$$

3.

$$127 = 10^x$$

To solve, take the common log *of both sides*:

$$\log 127 = \log(10^x)$$

$$\log 127 = x \log 10$$

$$2.1 \approx x(1)$$

$$x \approx 2.1$$

4.

$$\frac{1}{2}e^x = 10$$

$$e^x = 2(10) = 20$$

To solve, take ln *of both sides*:

$$\ln(e^x) = \ln 20$$

$$x \ln e = \ln 20$$

$$x(1) = 2.996$$

$$x \approx 3$$

5.
$$10^{2x} = 50$$

To solve, take log of both sides:

$$\log(10^{2x}) = \log 50$$
$$2x \log 10 = \log 50$$
$$(2x)(1) = 1.699$$
$$x = \frac{1}{2}(1.699) \approx 0.85$$

6.
$$(0.5)^x = 10$$

To solve, take either ln or log of both sides:

$$\ln(0.5)^x = \ln 10$$
$$x \ln(0.5) = \ln 10$$
$$x(-0.693) = 2.303$$
$$x \approx \frac{2.303}{-0.693} \approx -3.32$$

7.
$$(0.5)^{2x} = 18$$

To solve, take either ln or log of both sides:

$$\log(0.5)^{2x} = \log 18$$
$$(2x) \log 0.5 = \log 18$$
$$(2x)(-0.301) \approx 1.255$$
$$2x \approx \frac{1.255}{-0.301} \approx -4.169$$

P

8.

$$5(0.5)^x = 0.25$$

$$(0.5)^x = \frac{1}{5}(0.25) = 0.05$$

To solve, take either ln *or* log *of both sides*:

$$\ln(0.5)^x = \ln 0.05$$

$$x \ln(0.5) = \ln(0.05)$$

$$x(-0.693) = -2.996$$

$$x = \frac{-2.996}{-0.693} \approx 4.3$$

Worksheet 2-5: Linear and Semi-Log Graphs

I.

1. Using the equation: V = I(10), the completed table becomes:

I	0	5	10	20
V	0	50	100	200

2. Note: the vertical axis should extend from 0 to 500 volts. This is a linear graph.

3a. This graph represents a direct relationship between V and I.

b. when I = 35A, V = 350 volts

when I = 42A, V = 420 volts

c. when V = 15 volts, I = 1.5A

when V = 38 volts, I = 3.8A

d. slope = 10; this is the magnitude of the resistance

4a. This graph represents an indirect relationship between pressure and volume

b. when V = 0, P = 90 Pa

when V = 40 cc, P = 14 Pa

c. when P = 85 Pa, V ≈ 2 cc

when P = 20 Pa, V = 37 cc

d. y = mx + b

p = (-1.9)V + 90

note: $slope = m = \dfrac{Y_2 - Y_1}{X_2 - X_1}$

$= \dfrac{52-90}{20-0} = -1.9$

y-intercept = 90 Pa

II.

1.

Pb Thickness (mm)	Intensity Transmitted (I)	Fraction Transmitted (I/I_o)	% Transmitted $(I/I_o$ x 100%)	% Attenuated
0.0 mm	3700 (I_o)	$\frac{3700}{3700} = 1.0$	100%	0%
0.1 mm	2937	$\frac{2937}{3700} = 0.7$	79.4%	20.6%
0.2 mm	2331	$\frac{2331}{3700} = 0.6$	63%	37%
0.4 mm	1468		39.7%	60.3%
0.6 mm	925	$\frac{1468}{3700} = 0.3$	25%	75%
		$\frac{925}{3700} = 0.2$		

2. This is not a linear relationship.

3. When plotted on semi-log graph paper, the graph is linear.

4a. When transmission = 15%, thickness ≈ 0.82 mm

b. When transmission = 78%, thickness ≈ 0.11 mm

c. When transmission = 50%, thickness ≈ 0.3 mm

d. When thickness = 0.5 mm, transmission = 31.5% and attenuation = 68.5%

Worksheet 2-6: Areas and Volumes

I.   Area Calculations

1.
$A = l \times w$

$= (4\ cm)(6\ cm) = 24\ cm^2$

155

2.

$$A = 24\,cm^2 \times \left(\frac{1\ in}{2.54\ cm}\right)^2 \times \left(\frac{1\ ft}{12\ in}\right)^2$$

$$= \left(24 \times \frac{1}{6.45} \times \frac{1}{144}\right) ft^2$$

$$\approx 2.58 \times 10^{-2}\ ft^2$$

3.

$$A = \Pi r^2$$

$$= (3.14)(10\ cm)^2$$

$$= 314\ cm^2$$

$$A = \Pi r^2$$

$$= (3.14)(100\ mm)^2$$

$$= 3.14 \times 10^4\ mm^2$$

II. Volume Calculations

1.

$$V = l \times w \times h$$

$$= 10\,mm \times 5\,cm \times 8\,cm$$

$$= 1\,cm \times 5\,cm \times 8\,cm$$

$$= 40\ cm^3$$

2.

$$V = 40\,cm^3 \times \left(\frac{1\ in}{2.54\,cm}\right)^3$$

$$\approx \left(40 \times \frac{1}{16.39}\right) in^3$$

$$\approx 2.4\ in^3$$

3.

$$V = \Pi r^2 h$$

$$= (3.14)(5\,cm)^2(25\,cm)$$

$$= 1962.5\ cm^3$$

III. Calculations Involving Volume

1.

$$\rho = \frac{M}{V}$$

$$V = \frac{M}{\rho}$$

$$V = \frac{180 \; gm}{13.6 \frac{gm}{cc}}$$

$$V \approx 13.2 cc$$

2.

$$\rho = \frac{M}{V}$$

$$M = \rho V$$

$$M = (11.3 \frac{gm}{cc})(30 cc)$$

$$M = 339 gms.$$

3.

$$\rho = \frac{M}{V}$$

$$\rho = \frac{314.4 \; gms}{40 \; cc} = 7.86 \frac{gm}{cc}$$

The metal is **iron**.

Worksheet 2-7: Units and Unit Conversions

I.

1. $0.1 \; m = 1 \times 10^{-1} \; m$

2. $10 \; cm = 1 \times 10^{1} \; cm$

3. $8 \times 10^{-2} \; m$

4. $15 \times 10^{-3} \; kg = 1.5 \times 10^{-2} \; kg$

5. $200 \times 10^{-3} \; mg = 2 \times 10^{-1} \; mg$

6. $150 \times 10^{-3} \; kg = 1.5 \times 10^{-1} \; kg$

7. $630 \times 10^{3} \; gm = 6.3 \times 10^{5} \; gm$

8. $10 \times 10^{3} \; mcg = 1 \times 10^{4} \; mcg$

9. $500 \times 10^{-6} \times 10^{-3}$ kg $= 5 \times 10^2 \times 10^{-9}$ kg $= 5 \times 10^{-7}$ kg

10. 10×10^{-3} seconds $= 1 \times 10^{-2}$ seconds

11. 50×10^3 ms $= 5 \times 10^4$ ms

12. $40 \times 10^3 \mu s = 4 \times 10^4 \mu s$

13. $5 \times 10^3 \times 10^3$ mm $= 5 \times 10^6$ mm

14. 20×10^{-6} seconds $= 2 \times 10^{-5}$ seconds

15. 25×10^6 mcg $= 2.5 \times 10^7$ mcg

II. Unit Conversions - Dimensional Analysis

1.

$$10 \ m \times \frac{10^2 cm}{1m} \times \frac{1 \ in}{2.54 \ cm} \times \frac{1 \ ft}{12 \ in}$$

$$= \left(10 \times 10^2 \times \frac{1}{2.54} \times \frac{1}{12} \right) ft.$$

$$\approx 32.8 \ ft = 3.28 \times 10^1 \ ft$$

2.

$$10^2 \ in \times \frac{2.54}{1 \ in} \times \frac{10 \ mm}{1 \ cm}$$

$$= (10^2 \times 2.54 \times 10) \ mm$$

$$= 2.54 \times 10^3 \ mm$$

3.

$$20 \ cm \times \frac{1 \ in}{2.54 \ cm} \times \frac{1 \ ft}{12 \ in} \times \frac{1 \ yd}{3 \ ft}$$

$$= \left(20 \times \frac{1}{2.54} \times \frac{1}{12} \times \frac{1}{3} \right) yd$$

$$\approx 0.22 \ yd = 2.2 \times 10^{-1} \ yd$$

4.

$$2 \times 10^3 \ mcg \times \frac{1 \ gm}{10^6 \ mcg} \times \frac{1 \ kg}{10^3 \ gm} \times \frac{2.2 \ lb}{1 \ kg}$$

$$= (2 \times 10^3 \times 10^{-6} \times 10^{-3} \times 2.2) \ lbs$$

$$= 4.4 \times 10^{-6} \ lbs$$

5.

$$150 \ ms \times \frac{1 \ sec}{10^3 \ ms} \times \frac{1 \ min}{60 \ sec} \times \frac{1 \ hr}{60 \ min}$$

$$= (150 \times 10^{-3} \times \frac{1}{60} \times \frac{1}{60}) \ hr$$

$$= 4.2 \times 10^{-5} \ hr$$

6.

$$200 \ volts \times \frac{1 \ kilovolt}{10^3 \ volts}$$

$$= (2 \times 10^2 \times 10^{-3}) \ kV$$

$$= 2 \times 10^{-1} \ kV$$

7.

$$20 \ min \times \frac{60 \ sec}{1 \ min} \times \frac{10^6 \mu s}{1 \ sec}$$

$$= (20 \times 60 \times 10^6) \ \mu s$$

$$= 1.2 \times 10^9 \ \mu s$$

8.

$$70 \ mm \times \frac{1 \ cm}{10 \ mm} \times \frac{1 \ in}{2.54 \ cm}$$

$$= \left(70 \times 10^{-1} \times \frac{1}{2.54}\right) in$$

$$\approx 2.8 \ in$$

9.

$$10 \ km \times \frac{10^3 \ m}{1 \ km} \times \frac{10^2 cm}{1 \ m} \times \frac{1 \ in}{2.54 \ cm} \times \frac{1 \ ft}{12 \ in} \times \frac{1 \ mile}{5280 \ ft}$$

$$= \left(10 \times 10^3 \times 10^2 \times \frac{1}{2.54} \times \frac{1}{12} \times \frac{1}{5280}\right) mile$$

$$\approx 6.2 \ miles$$

10.

$$400 \ gm \times \frac{1 \ kg}{10^3 \ gm} \times \frac{2.2 \ lbs}{1 \ kg} \times \frac{16 \ oz}{1 \ lb}$$

$$= (400 \times 10^{-3} \times 2.2 \times 16) \ oz$$

$$\approx 1.4 \times 10^1 \ oz$$

11.

$$200 \text{ } millivolts \times \frac{10^3 \text{ } microvolts}{1 \text{ } millivolt}$$

$$= (200 \times 10^3) \text{ } microvolts$$

$$= 2 \times 10^5 \text{ } microvolts$$

12.

$$5A \times \frac{10^3 mA}{1A}$$

$$= 5 \times 10^3 \text{ } mA$$

13.

$$10 \text{ } in \times \frac{2.54 \text{ } cm}{1 \text{ } in} \times \frac{1 \text{ } m}{10^2 \text{ } cm} \times \frac{1 \text{ Å}}{10^{-10} \text{ } m}$$

$$= (10 \times 2.54 \times 10^{-2} \times 10^{10}) \text{ Å}$$

$$\approx 2.5 \times 10^9 \text{ Å}$$

14.

$$0.1\text{Å} \times \frac{10^{-10} m}{1\text{Å}} \times \frac{10^2 \text{ } cm}{1 \text{ } m} \times \frac{1 \text{ } in}{2.54 \text{ } cm}$$

$$= \left(0.1 \times 10^{-10} \times 10^2 \times \frac{1}{2.54}\right) \text{ } in$$

$$\approx 3.9 \times 10^{-10} \text{ } in$$

15.

$$10^{-3} \text{ } cm \times \frac{1 \text{ } m}{10^2 \text{ } cm} \times \frac{1\text{Å}}{10^{-10} m}$$

$$= (10^{-3} \times 10^{-2} \times 10^{10}) \text{ Å}$$

$$= 1 \times 10^5 \text{ Å}$$

Worksheet 2-8: Velocity and Acceleration

I. Velocity Calculations

1.
   Given: $\Delta d = 80\ cm = 0.8m$

   $\Delta t = 400\ \mu s = 400 \times 10^{-6}s = 4 \times 10^{-4}s$

   $$V = \frac{\Delta d}{\Delta t}$$

   $$= \frac{0.8m}{4 \times 10^{-4}s}$$

   $$= 2 \times 10^3\ \frac{m}{s}$$

2.
   Given: $V = 1.5\ \frac{km}{s}$

   $\Delta d = 50\ cm = 5 \times 10^{-4}km$

   $$V = \frac{\Delta d}{\Delta t}$$

   $$\Delta t = \frac{\Delta d}{V} = \frac{5 \times 10^{-4}\ km}{1.5\frac{km}{s}} \approx 3.3 \times 10^{-4}sec\ or\ 0.33\ ms$$

3.
   Given: $V = 1.5 \times 10^8 \frac{m}{s}$

   $\Delta t = 3.3 \times 10^{-9}sec$

   $$V = \frac{\Delta d}{\Delta t}$$

   $$\Delta d = (v)(\Delta t)$$

   $$= \left(1.5 \times 10^8 \frac{m}{s}\right)(3.3 \times 10^{-9}sec)$$

   $$\approx 4.95 \times 10^{-1}m$$

161

4.

$$\text{Given: } V = c = 3 \times 10^8 \frac{m}{s}$$

$$\Delta d = 1 \text{ } mile \approx 1.6 \times 10^3 m$$

$$V = \frac{\Delta d}{\Delta t}$$

$$\Delta t = \frac{\Delta d}{V}$$

$$= \frac{1.6 \times 10^3 m}{3 \times 10^8 \frac{m}{s}}$$

$$\approx 5.3 \times 10^{-6} \sec (or \text{ } 5.3 \mu s)$$

II. Acceleration Calculations

1.

$$\text{Given: } v_i = 150 \frac{m}{s}$$

$(V_i = \text{ initial velocity}$
$V_f = \text{ final velocity})$

$$v_f = 2000 \frac{m}{s}$$

$$\Delta v = v_f - v_i = 2000 \frac{m}{s} - 150 \frac{m}{s} = 1850 \frac{m}{s}$$

$$\Delta t = 0.8 \sec$$

$$a = \frac{\Delta v}{\Delta t}$$

2.

$$= \frac{1850 \frac{m}{s}}{0.8 s}$$

$$= 2312.5 \frac{m}{s^2} \text{ } (or \text{ } \sim 2.3 \times 10^3 \frac{m}{s^2}$$

Given: $v_i = 120\frac{m}{s}$

$\ \ v_f = 155\frac{m}{s}$

$\ \ \Delta v = v_f - v_i = 155\frac{m}{s} - 120\frac{m}{s} = 35\frac{m}{s}$

$\ \ a = 5\frac{m}{s^2}$

$\ \ a = \frac{\Delta v}{\Delta t}$

$\Delta t = \frac{\Delta v}{a}$

$$= \frac{35\ \frac{m}{s}}{5\frac{m}{s^2}} = 7\ sec$$

3.

Given: $v_i = 0$ (at rest)

$\ \ v_f = 39.2\frac{m}{s}$

$\ \ \Delta v = v_f - v_i = 39.2\frac{m}{s}$

$\ \ \Delta t = 4\ sec$

$\ \ a = \frac{\Delta v}{\Delta t}$

$\ \ a = \frac{39.2\frac{m}{s}}{4s}$

$\ \ a = 9.8\frac{m}{s^2}$

4.   *Given:* $v_i = 0$ (*at rest*)

$$v_f = 2 \times 10^8 \frac{m}{s}$$

$$\Delta v = v_f - v_i = 2 \times 10^8 \frac{m}{s}$$

$$\Delta t = 5 \, \mu s = 5 \times 10^{-6} \, sec$$

$$a = \frac{\Delta v}{\Delta t}$$

$$a = \frac{2 \times 10^8 \frac{m}{s}}{5 \times 10^{-6} sec}$$

$$= 0.4 \times 10^{14} \frac{m}{s^2}$$

$$= 4 \times 10^{13} \frac{m}{s^2}$$

Worksheet 2-9: Force, Momentum and Energy

I.

    1. d

    2. c

    3. b

    4. d

    5. a

    6. b

    7. c

    8. a

    9. a

   10. c

II.

    1.

$$10^3 eV \times \frac{1 MeV}{10^6 eV} = 10^{-3} MeV$$

2.

$$10^2 keV \times \frac{10^3 eV}{1 keV} = 10^5 eV$$

3.

$$50 \ keV \times \frac{1 MeV}{10^3 keV} = 50 \times 10^{-3} MeV = 5 \times 10^{-2} MeV$$

4.

$$8 \times 10^4 eV \times \frac{1 MeV}{10^6 eV} = 8 \times 10^{-2} MeV$$

5.

$$10 keV \times \frac{10^3 eV}{1 keV} = 10^4 eV$$

6.

$$10^2 eV \times \frac{1 keV}{10^3 eV} = 10^{-1} keV$$

7.

$$250 \ MeV \times \frac{10^3 keV}{1 \ MeV} = 2.5 \times 10^5 keV$$

8.

$$50 \ MeV \times \frac{10^6 eV}{1 \ MeV} = 5 \times 10^7 \ eV$$

9.

$$0.25 \ MeV \times \frac{10^3 keV}{1 \ MeV} = 0.25 \times 10^3 \ keV = 2.5 \times 10^2 keV$$

10.

$$0.50 \ keV \times \frac{10^3 eV}{1 \ keV} = 0.50 \times 10^3 \ eV = 5 \times 10^2 eV$$

III.

1.

$$F = ma$$

$$= (9.1 \times 10^{-31} kg)\left(5 \times 10^2 \frac{m}{s^2}\right)$$

$$\approx 4.6 \times 10^{-28} \ Newtons$$

2.

$$F = ma \qquad \left(but\ m = \frac{weight}{g} = \frac{64\ lbs}{32\ \frac{ft}{s^2}} = 2\ slugs \right)$$

$$20\ lbs = (2\ slugs)(a)$$

$$a = \frac{20\ lbs}{2\ slugs} = 10\ \frac{ft}{s^2}$$

3.

$$KE = \frac{1}{2}mv^2$$

$$= \left(\frac{1}{2}\right)(2 \times 10^{-2} kg)(5 \times 10^2 \frac{m}{s})^2$$

$$= 2.5 \times 10^3 joules$$

$$KE = 2.5 \times 10^3 joules \times \frac{1\ eV}{1.6 \times 10^{-19} joules}$$

$$\approx 1.56 \times 10^{22} eV = 1.56 \times 10^{16} MeV$$

4.

$$KE = \frac{1}{2}mv^2$$

$$v = \sqrt{\frac{2\ KE}{m}}$$

$$v = \sqrt{\frac{(2)(0.01\ joule)}{2 \times 10^{-3}\ kg}}$$

$$= \sqrt{1 \times 10^1 \frac{m^2}{s^2}}$$

$$\approx 3.2 \frac{m}{s}$$

5a. mass of 4 hydrogen atoms = $4 \times 1.673 \times 10^{-27} kg$
$$= 6.692 \times 10^{-27} kg$$

mass difference = $(6.692 \times 10^{-27} kg) - (6.646 \times 10^{-27} kg)$
$$= 4.6 \times 10^{-29} kg$$

energy liberated = mc^2
$$= (4.6 \times 10^{-29} kg)(3 \times 10^8\ m/s)^2$$
$$= 4.14 \times 10^{-12}\ joules$$

b.

$$\text{no of He atoms} = \frac{10^7 \text{joules}}{4.14 \times 10^{-12} \frac{joules}{atom}}$$

$$\approx 2.4 \times 10^{18} \quad \text{He atoms}$$

6.

$$E = 50 \text{ keV} \times \frac{10^3 eV}{1 \text{ keV}} \times \frac{1.6 \times 10^{-19} joules}{1 \text{ eV}}$$

$$= 8 \times 10^{-15} joules$$

$$KE = \frac{1}{2}mv^2$$

$$v = \sqrt{\frac{2 \text{ } KE}{m}}$$

$$= \sqrt{\frac{2 \times 8 \times 10^{-15} \text{ joules}}{9.1 \times 10^{-31} kg}}$$

$$\approx \sqrt{1.76 \times 10^{16} \frac{m}{s}}$$

$$\approx 1.3 \times 10^8 \frac{m}{s}$$

7.

$$KE = \frac{1}{2}mv^2$$

$$= \frac{1}{2}(9.1 \times 10^{-31} kg)\left(10^6 \frac{m}{s}\right)^2$$

$$\approx 4.6 \times 10^{-19} \text{ joules}$$

$$E = 4.6 \times 10^{-19} joules \times \frac{1 \text{ eV}}{1.6 \times 10^{-19} joules}$$

$$\approx 2.9 \text{ eV}$$

Worksheet 2-10: Work and Power

I.

    1. c

    2. d

3. a

4. b

5. d

6. a

7. b

8. d

9. a

10. b

II.

1.

$$P = \frac{W}{t}$$

$$W = P \times t$$

$$= (10^3 watts)(1800 \ sec.)$$

$$= 1.8 \times 10^6 joules$$

2.

$$P = \frac{W}{t} = \frac{F \times d}{t}$$

$$= \frac{(10^4 N)(10^2 m)}{5 \ sec}$$

$$= 2 \times 10^5 \ watts$$

3.

$$P = \frac{W}{t}$$

$$t = \frac{W}{P}$$

$$= \frac{2 \times 10^3 joules}{1 \times 10^2 \ watts}$$

$$= 2 \times 10 \ sec \quad or \quad 20 \ sec.$$

4.

$$P = \frac{W}{t}$$

Work(or Energy) = *Power* × *time*

= *(kilowatt)(hour)*

*Therefore the kilowatt-hour is a unit of **energy**.*

Worksheet 2-11: Physics Review: Flux and Intensity

1. b
2. a
3. a
4. a
5. a
6. c
7. b
8. c
9. d
10. a
11. a
12. a

Worksheet 2-12: Physics Review: Methods of Heat Transfer

1. b
2. d
3. a
4. c
5. a
6. b
7. b

8. b

Worksheet 3-1: Atomic Structure

I.

1. b

2. a

3. b

4. c   (N = A−Z = 32−15 = 17)

5. b   (A = N+Z = 12+30 = 42)

6. d

7. a

8. d

9. b

10. b

11. c $(E = E_N−E_K = -0.025 \text{ keV} + 10 \text{ keV} = 9.975 \text{ keV})$

12. d

13. a   (E is greater than 33−35 eV)

14. a
$$\lambda = \frac{12.4}{9.975 \ keV} = 1.24 \text{ Å}$$

15. b   (1.24 Å is less than 4000 Å − 7000 Å)

16. b
$$\left(\lambda = \frac{12.4}{0.002 \ keV} = 6200 \text{ Å}\right)$$

17. a (6200 Å falls between the visible wavelength limits of 4000 Å − 7000 Å)

18. d

19. c

20. b

II.

1. 15 protons

2. 32-15 = 17 neutrons

3. 15 electrons (in order for the atom to be electrically neutral, the atom must have the same number of electrons as protons)

4. isotopes

5. 1/2000

Worksheet 3-2: Nuclear Structure

1. a

2. c

3. d

4. c

5. a   (lower binding energy per nucleon)

6. c

7. a

8. d

9. a

10. a

Worksheet 3-3: Radiation Characteristics and Properties

I.

1. b

2. c

3. a

4. c

5. c

6. a

7. b

8. d

9. a

10. c

11. b

12. c

13. d

14. c

15. b

II. 1. positrons: +1

   negatrons: -1

   alphas: +2

   gamma: 0

   x-rays: 0

2. bremsstrahlung

   "braking radiation"

3. For a 60 keV photon:

$$\lambda \text{ (Å)} = \frac{12.4}{E(keV)}$$

$$= \frac{12.4}{60 \ keV} \approx 0.21\text{Å}$$

For a 100 keV photon:

$$\lambda \text{ (Å)} = \frac{12.4}{100 \ keV} = 0.124\text{Å}$$

Worksheet 3-4: Properties of Waves

I.

    1. d

    2. c

    3. a

    4. d

    5. c

    6. b

    7. a

    8. b

    9. a

    10. d

II.

    1.

$$v = f\lambda$$

$$\lambda = \frac{v}{f}$$

$$= \frac{2.25 \times 10^8 \frac{m}{s}}{3 \times 10^{10}\ Hz}$$

$$= 7.5 \times 10^{-3} m \quad or\ 7.5\ mm$$

    2a.

$$c = f\lambda$$

$$\lambda = \frac{c}{f}$$

$$= \frac{3 \times 10^8 \frac{m}{s}}{4.3 \times 10^{14}\ Hz}$$

$$= 6.977 \times 10^{-7} m$$

$$or\ 6.977 \times 10^{-7} m \times \frac{1\overset{\circ}{A}}{10^{-10}m} = 6977\overset{\circ}{A}$$

b.

$$E(keV) = \frac{12.4}{\lambda(\text{Å})}$$

$$= \frac{12.4}{6977\text{Å}} \approx 1.78 \times 10^{-3} keV \text{ or } 1.78 \text{ eV}$$

c. This photon is non-ionizing since it has an energy less than 33-35 eV.

3. All photons travel at the same speed in air, 3×10^8 m/s.

4a.

$$E(keV) = \frac{12.4}{8500\text{Å}}$$

$$\approx 1.46 \times 10^{-3} keV \text{ or } 1.46 \text{ eV} \quad (non\text{-}ionizing)$$

b.

$$0.01m \times \frac{1\text{Å}}{10^{-10}m} = 10^8\text{Å}$$

$$E(keV) = \frac{12.4}{10^8\text{Å}} = 12.4 \times 10^{-8} keV$$

$$\text{or } 12.4 \times 10^{-5} eV \quad (non\text{-}ionizing)$$

c.

$$3.125m \times \frac{1\text{Å}}{10^{-10}m} = 3.125 \times 10^{10}\text{Å}$$

$$E(keV) = \frac{12.4}{3.125 \times 10^{10}\text{Å}} \approx 3.97 \times 10^{-10} keV$$

$$\text{or } 3.97 \times 10^{-7} eV \quad (non\text{-}ionizing)$$

Worksheet 3-5: Inverse Square Law

1.
$$I_1 d_1^2 = I_2 d_2^2$$

$$\left(40\frac{mR}{hr}\right)(10\ cm)^2 = I_2(15\ cm)^2$$

$$I_2 = \left(40\frac{mR}{hr}\right)\left(\frac{10\ cm}{15\ cm}\right)^2$$

$$= \left(40\frac{mR}{hr}\right)(0.44)$$

$$\approx 17.8\frac{mR}{hr}$$

2.
$$I_1 d_1^2 = I_2 d_2^2$$

$$\left(25\frac{mR}{hr}\right)(3\ ft)^2 = \left(2\frac{mR}{hr}\right)(d_2^2)$$

$$d_2^2 = \frac{\left(25\frac{mR}{hr}\right)(9\,ft^2)}{2\frac{mR}{hr}}$$

$$= 112.5\ ft^2$$

$$d_2 \approx 10.6\ ft$$

3.
$$I_1 d_1^2 = I_2 d_2^2$$

$$\left(200\frac{mR}{hr}\right)(5\ m)^2 = I_2(1.5m)^2$$

$$I_2 = \left(200\frac{mR}{hr}\right)\left(\frac{5m}{1.5m}\right)^2$$

$$= \left(200\frac{mR}{hr}\right)(3.3)^2$$

$$\approx 2178\frac{mR}{hr}$$

4.
$$I_1 d_1^2 = i_2 d_2^2$$

$$I_0(8m)^2 = (0.3I_0)(d_2^2)$$

$$d_2^2 = \frac{(I_0)(8m)^2}{(0.3\ I_0)}$$

$$= 213.3\ m^2$$

$$d_2 \approx 14.6\ m$$

5.

$$I_1 d_1^2 = I_2 d_2^2$$

$$(I_0)(8m)^2 = (0.5 I_0)(d_2^2)$$

$$d_2^2 = \frac{(I_0)(8m)^2}{(0.5\ I_0)}$$

$$= 128\ m^2$$

$$d_2 \approx 11.3\ m$$

Worksheet 4-1: Static Electricity

I. 1. d

2. a

3. a

4. b

5. b

6. a

7. c

8. d

9. c

10. a

11. a

II. 1.

$$F_E = K\frac{q_1 q_2}{d^2}$$

$$= \left(9 \times 10^9\ \frac{N\text{-}m^2}{c^2}\right)\frac{(1.6 \times 10^{-19}C)^2}{(10^{-10}m)^2}$$

$$\approx 2.3 \times 10^{-8}\ N,\ repulsive$$

2a.

$$F_E = K\frac{q_1 q_2}{d^2}$$

$$= \left(9 \times 10^9\ \frac{N\text{-}m^2}{c^2}\right)\frac{(-1.6 \times 10^{-19}C)(1.6 \times 10^{-19}C)}{(5.3 \times 10^{-11}m)^2}$$

$$\approx -8.2 \times 10^{-9}\ N$$

The negative sign implies this is an **attractive** force.

b.

$$F_G = G\frac{m_1 m_2}{d^2}$$

$$= \left(6.7 \times 10^{-11}\frac{N\text{-}m^2}{c^2}\right)\frac{(9.1 \times 10^{-31}kg)\,(1.67 \times 10^{-27}kg)}{(5.3 \times 10^{-11}m)^2}$$

$$\approx 3.6 \times 10^{-47}\ N$$

$$\frac{F_E}{F_G} = \frac{8.2 \times 10^{-9}N}{3.6 \times 10^{-47}N} \approx 2.3 \times 10^{38}$$

The above ratio implies that the electric force (F_E) is some 10^{38} times greater than the gravitational force (F_G). Thus the F_E is the more dominant force in holding the electron to the atom.

Worksheet 4-2: Current, Voltage, and Resistance

I.
1. b
2. d
3. b
4. b
5. c
6. b
7. d
8. a
9. b
10. c

II.
1.

$$number\ of\ electrons = \frac{total\ excess\ charge}{charge\ per\ electron}$$

$$= \frac{-1\ coulomb}{-1.6 \times 10^{-19}\frac{C}{e}}$$

$$= 6.25 \times 10^{18}\ electrons$$

2.

$$number\ of\ electrons\ removed = \frac{+0.20C}{1.6 \times 10^{-19}\frac{C}{e}}$$

$$= 1.25 \times 10^{18}\ electrons$$

3.

$$\text{current} = \frac{\text{charge}}{\text{time}}$$

$$= \frac{(10^6)(1.6 \times 10^{-19}C)}{1 \text{ sec}}$$

$$= 1.6 \times 10^{-13} \text{ amps}$$

4.

$$I = \frac{q}{t}$$

$$q = (I)(t)$$

$$= (1 \text{ amp})(1 \text{ msec})$$

$$= \left(1\frac{C}{s}\right)(1 \times 10^{-3}\text{sec})$$

$$= 10^{-3}C$$

$$\text{number of electrons} = \frac{\text{charge}}{\text{charge per electron}}$$

$$= \frac{10^{-3}C}{1.6 \times 10^{-19}\frac{C}{e}}$$

$$= 6.25 \times 10^{15} \text{ electrons must flow through}$$
the wire each msec.

5.

$$V = IR$$

$$I = \frac{V}{R}$$

$$= \frac{120 \text{ v}}{5 \times 10^4 \Omega}$$

$$= 2.4 \times 10^{-3} \text{ amps or } 2.4 \text{ mA}$$

6.

$$V = IR$$

$$= (5.5A)(1500\Omega)$$

$$= 8250 \text{ volts}$$

7.

$$V = IR$$

$$R = \frac{V}{I}$$

$$= \frac{110 \text{ volts}}{3.2 \times 10^{-3}\text{amps}}$$

$$\approx 3.4 \times 10^4 \Omega$$

8.

$$V = IR$$

$$= (5 \times 10^{-3}A)(10^3\Omega)$$

$$= 5 \ volts$$

9.

$$V = IR$$

$$R = \frac{V}{I}$$

$$= \frac{120 \ volts}{1.5 \ amps} = 80\Omega$$

Worksheet 4-3: DC Circuits

1. a.
$$R_T = 5\Omega + 10\Omega + 4\Omega + 2\Omega = 21\Omega$$

   b.
$$V = IR$$

$$I = \frac{V}{R}$$

$$= \frac{20 \ volts}{21 \ \Omega} \approx 0.95 \ amps$$

2. a.
$$\frac{1}{R_T} = \frac{1}{3\Omega} + \frac{1}{8\Omega} + \frac{1}{4\Omega}$$

$$= \frac{8}{24\Omega} + \frac{3}{24\Omega} + \frac{6}{24\Omega}$$

$$= \frac{17}{24\Omega}$$

$$R_T \approx \frac{24\Omega}{17} \approx 1.4\Omega$$

   b.

For parallel branch: $\frac{1}{R_T} = \frac{1}{6\Omega} + \frac{1}{4\Omega}$

$$= \frac{2}{12\Omega} + \frac{3}{12\Omega}$$

$$= \frac{5}{12\Omega}$$

$$R_T = \frac{12\Omega}{5} = 2.4\Omega$$

Then for entire circuit: $R_T = 4\Omega + 2.4\Omega + 3\Omega$

$$= 9.4\Omega$$

c. Consider each parallel branch separately, then just add:

$$\frac{1}{R_1} = \frac{1}{2\Omega} + \frac{1}{10\Omega}$$

$$= \frac{5}{10\Omega} + \frac{1}{10\Omega}$$

$$= \frac{6}{10\Omega}$$

$$R_1 = \frac{10\Omega}{6} \approx 1.7\Omega$$

$$\frac{1}{R_2} = \frac{1}{5\Omega} + \frac{1}{4\Omega}$$

$$= \frac{4}{20\Omega} + \frac{5}{20\Omega}$$

$$= \frac{9}{20\Omega}$$

$$R_2 = \frac{20\Omega}{9} \approx 2.2\Omega$$

$$R_T = R_1 + R_2$$

$$= 1.7\Omega + 2.2\Omega$$

$$= 3.9\Omega$$

3.a.

$$R_T = R_1 + R_2 + R_3$$

$$= 2\Omega + 4\Omega + 6\Omega$$

$$= 12\Omega$$

b.

$$V_T = I_T R_T$$

$$I_T = \frac{V_T}{R_T} = \frac{12v}{12\Omega} = 1 \ amp$$

c. 1 amp flows through each resistance since current is constant in series circuits.

d.

$$V_1 = I_1R_1$$

$$= (1A)(2\Omega) = 2 \; volts$$

$$V_2 = I_2R_2$$

$$= (1A)(4\Omega) = 4 \; volts$$

$$V_3 = I_3R_3$$

$$= (1A)(6\Omega) = 6 \; volts$$

$$V_T = 2v + 4v + 6v = 12 \; volts$$

4.a.

$$\frac{1}{R_T} = \frac{1}{3\Omega} + \frac{1}{4\Omega} + \frac{1}{12\Omega}$$

$$= \frac{4}{12\Omega} + \frac{3}{12\Omega} + \frac{1}{12\Omega}$$

$$= \frac{8}{12\Omega}$$

$$R_T = \frac{12\Omega}{8} = 1.5\Omega$$

b.

$$V_T = I_TR_T$$

$$I_T = \frac{V_T}{R_T} = \frac{12v}{1.5\Omega} = 8 \; amp$$

c. The voltage across R_1, R_2, and R_3 is 12 volts since voltage is constant in parallel circuits.

d.

$$V = IR, \text{ so } I = \frac{V}{R}$$

$$I_1 = \frac{V_1}{R_1}$$

$$= \frac{12v}{3\Omega} = 4 \text{ amps}$$

$$I_2 = \frac{V_2}{R_2}$$

$$= \frac{12v}{4\Omega} = 3 \text{ amps}$$

$$I_3 = \frac{V_3}{R_3}$$

$$= \frac{12v}{12\Omega} = 1 \text{ amp}$$

When these currents are totalled, they give the total current in the circuit (i.e., 8 amps)

e. R_T will always be less than the smallest of the individual resistances in the parallel portion of the circuit.

Worksheet 4-4: AC Rectification

I. 1. d
    2. b
    3. a
    4. b
    5. a
    6. b
    7. c
    8. c
    9. b
    10. d
    11. c
    12. c
    13. b
    14. c
    15. b

II. In a full-wave rectified system, 1/2 cycle occurs every 1/120 second. Therefore, the number of half-cycles that occur will be:

1.

$$\frac{1\ second}{\frac{1}{120}\ second} = 120\ half\ cycles$$

2.

$$\frac{0.500\ second}{\frac{1}{120} second} = 60\ half\ cycles$$

3.

$$\frac{\frac{1}{120}\ second}{\frac{1}{120} second} = 1\ half\ cycle$$

4.

$$\frac{0.050\ second}{\frac{1}{120}\ second} = 6\ half\ cycles$$

5.

$$\frac{.008\ second}{\frac{1}{120}\ second} = 0.96\ half\ cycle$$

III. 1. single phase, unrectified

2. single phase, full-wave rectified

3. three phase, full-wave rectified

4. single phase, half-wave rectified

5. three phase, unrectified

IV. 1. 100% (voltage drops to zero)

2.

$$\frac{80V-70V}{80V} \times 100\% = 12.5\%$$

3.

$$\frac{320V - 240V}{320V} \times 100\% = 25\%$$

Worksheet 5-1: Electromagnetic Effects

I.

1. current flow is to the left (i.e., opposite to the direction of electron flow)

2. current flow is to the right (i.e., in the same direction of positive charge movement)

II. Magnetic field lines travel from **North** to **South** outside the magnet.
Magnetic field lines travel from **South** to **North** inside the magnet.

III. Using the right hand rule:

1. thumb is positioned parallel and in the same direction of positive charge (p^+) flow; **B** lines travel out of the page above the wire and into the page below the wire

2. thumb is positioned parallel but opposite in direction to electron flow; **B** lines travel out of the page above the wire and into the page below the wire.

3. thumb is positioned parallel but opposite in direction to electron flow; **B** lines travel into the page above the wire and out the page below the wire

IV.

1. current flows from positive to negative terminal of battery; the current therefore flows up the outside of the coil

2. using the right hand rule, **B** lines inside the coil travel from right end of coil to the left end of coil; therefore right end of coil is S and left end is N

3. **B** lines travel from right to left inside the coil

V.

1. current flows down front side of coil; right end of coil is N, left end of coil is S; **B** field lines inside coil travel from left to right

2. current flows down front side of coil; right end of coil is N, left end of coil is S; **B** field lines inside coil travel from left to right

3. current flows up the front side of the coil; right end of coil is S, left end is N; **B** field lines inside coil travel from right to left

Worksheet 5-2: Electromagnetic Effects: Transformers

I.

1. left circuit is the primary (since it contains the power source), right circuit is the secondary; this is a step-down ($N_p > N_s$)

transformer

2. left circuit is the primary, right circuit is the secondary; this is a step-up $(N_p < N_s)$ transformer

II.

1.
$$\frac{I_p}{I_s} = \frac{N_s}{N_p}$$

$$\frac{2A}{I_s} = \frac{200}{800}$$

$$(800)(2A) = (200)(I_s)$$

$$I_s = \frac{(800)(2A)}{200} = 8A$$

2a.
$$\frac{V_s}{V_p} = \frac{N_s}{N_p}$$

$$\frac{10V}{V_p} = \frac{100}{600}$$

$$(100)(V_p) = (10v)(600)$$

$$V_p = \frac{(10v)(600)}{100} = 60 \; volts$$

b.
$$\frac{I_p}{I_s} = \frac{N_s}{N_p}$$

$$\frac{0.5A}{I_s} = \frac{100}{600}$$

$$(600)(0.5A) = (100)(I_s)$$

$$I_s = \frac{(600)(0.5A)}{100}$$

$$= 3A$$

c. this is a step down transformer $(N_p > N_s)$

3a.
$$\frac{V_s}{V_p} = \frac{N_s}{N_p}$$

$$\frac{V_s}{220v} = \frac{3000}{25}$$

$$(25)(V_s) = (3000)(220v)$$

$$V_s = \frac{(3000)(220v)}{25} = 26,400 \; volts$$

b.

$$\frac{I_p}{I_s} = \frac{N_s}{N_p}$$

$$\frac{2A}{I_s} = \frac{3000}{25}$$

$$(3000)(I_s) = (25)(2A)$$

$$I_s = \frac{(25)(2A)}{3000} \approx 0.017A \ or \ {\sim}17mA$$

c. This is a step-up transformer ($N_s > N_p$).

4a.

$$\frac{V_s}{V_p} = \frac{N_s}{N_p}$$

$$\frac{V_s}{100v} = \frac{150}{3500}$$

$$V_s = \frac{(150)(100V)}{3500} \approx 4.3 \ volts$$

b.

$$\frac{I_p}{I_s} = \frac{N_s}{N_p}$$

$$\frac{0.1A}{I_s} = \frac{150}{3500}$$

$$(150)(I_s) = (3500)(0.1A)$$

$$I_s = \frac{(3500)(0.1A)}{150} \approx 2.3A$$

5a.

$$\frac{V_s}{V_p} = \frac{N_s}{N_p}$$

$$\frac{80,000V}{55V} = \frac{N_s}{N_p}$$

$$\frac{N_s}{N_p} \approx 1454.5$$

b.

$$\frac{I_p}{I_s} = \frac{V_s}{V_p}$$

$$\frac{1A}{I_s} = \frac{80,000V}{55V}$$

$$(80,000V)(I_s) = (1A)(55V)$$

$$I_s = \frac{(1A)(55V)}{80,000V}$$

$$\approx 0.0007A \ or \ 0.7mA$$

c.

$$\frac{V_s}{V_p} = \frac{N_s}{N_p}$$

$$\frac{80,000V}{55V} = \frac{N_s}{25}$$

$$N_s = \frac{(25)(80,000\ V)}{55V} \approx 36,364\ turns$$

d. This is a step-up transformer (Ns > Np)

6a.

$$\frac{V_s}{V_p} = \frac{N_s}{N_p}$$

$$\frac{V_s}{220v} = \frac{75}{40}$$

$$(V_s) = \frac{(75)(220v)}{40} \approx 412.5\ volts$$

b.

$$\frac{V_s}{V_p} = \frac{N_s}{N_p}$$

$$\frac{V_s}{412.5v} = \frac{8000}{50}$$

$$(V_s) = \frac{(8000)(412.5v)}{50} = 66,000\ volts\ or\ 66\ kV$$

c. E_{MAX} = 66 keV

Worksheet 6-1: Heat Unit Calculations

1. HU = (kVp)(mA)(sec.)

    = (70 kVp)(200 mA)(0.1 sec)

    = 1400 HU

2. HU = (1.35)(kVp)(mA)(sec.)

    = (1.35)(80 kVp)(1000 mA)(0.01 sec)

    = 1080 HU

3. HU = (no. of exposures)(kVp)(mA)(sec)

    = (5)(80 kVp)(100 mA)(0.1 sec)

    = 4000 HU

4. HU = (no. of exposures)(1.41)(kVp)(mA)(sec)

    = (4)(1.41)(90 kVp)(800 mA)(0.001 sec)

    ≈ 406 HU

5. HU = (no. of exposures)(1.35)(kVp)(mA)(sec)

    = (10)(1.35)(70 kVp)(500 mA)(0.2 sec)

    = 94,500 HU

Worksheet 7-1: Checking A Timer (Spinning Top Technique)

I.

    1. Sketch should show all positive voltage pulses (no gaps); should be 120 pulses/sec

    2. Sketch should be same as #1 except there are 100 pulses/sec

    3. Sketch should show all positive pulses (no gaps) with 6 pulses each 1/60 sec (or 360 pulses/sec)

    4. Sketch should show all positive pulses (no gaps) with 12 pulses each 1/60 sec (or 720 pulses/sec)

II.

    1. Number of dots expected:
$$\frac{\frac{1}{20}\,sec}{\frac{1}{120}\,sec} = 6\ dots$$

Since only 6 dots were observed, the timer is too fast (i.e., it terminates the exposure too soon).

    2. Number of dots expected:
$$\frac{\frac{1}{20}\,sec}{\frac{1}{120}\,sec} = 6\ dots$$
Since 6 dots were observed, the timer is accurate

    3. Number of dots expected:
$$\frac{\frac{1}{20}\,sec}{\frac{1}{60}\,sec} = 3\ dots$$
Since 6 dots were observed, the timer is too slow (i.e., it terminates the exposure too late)

    4. Number of dots expected:
$$\frac{\frac{1}{30}\,sec}{\frac{1}{120}\,sec} = 4\ dots$$

Since 6 dots were observed, the timer is too slow (i.e., it terminates the exposure too late)

III.

    1.   Number of dots expected $= \left(\frac{1}{15}\sec\right)\left(\frac{120 \; dots}{\sec}\right)$

                                                     $= 8 \; dots$

    2.   Number of dots expected $= \left(\frac{1}{15}\sec\right)\left(\frac{60 \; dots}{\sec}\right)$

                                                       $= 4 \; dots$

Worksheet 8-1: Photon Interactions with Matter

I.

    1. d

    2. b

    3. c

    4. b

    5. d

    6. a

    7. a

    8. d

    9. a

  10. d

II.

    1. $E_{photon} = E_{binding} + E_{electron}$

        $30 \; keV = 28 \; keV + E_{electron}$

        $E_{electron} = 30 \; keV - 28 \; keV = 2 \; keV$

    2a.

        $E_{incident} = \frac{12.4}{\lambda \, (\text{Å})}$

                 $= \frac{12.4}{90 \; keV} \approx 0.1378\text{Å}$

    b. $\Delta\lambda = 0.0243 \, (1 - \cos 60°)$

           $= 0.0243 \, (1 - 0.5)$

           $\approx 0.0122\text{Å}$

    c. $\lambda' = \lambda + \Delta\lambda$

          $= 0.1378\text{Å} + 0.0122\text{Å}$

          $\approx 0.15\text{Å}$

d.

$$E' = \frac{12.4}{\lambda'(\text{Å})}$$

$$= \frac{12.4}{0.15\text{Å}} \approx 82.7\,keV$$

e.

$$E_{incident} = E_{SCAT} + E_{bind} + E_{e-}$$

$$90\ keV = 82.7\ keV + 0.5\ keV + E_{e}-$$

$$E_{e}- = 90\ keV - 83.2\ keV \approx 6.8\ keV$$

3.

$$E_{incident} = 1.02\ MeV + E_{e-} + E_{e+}$$

$$E_{e-} + E_{e+} = 18\ MeV - 1.02\ MeV = 16.98\ MeV$$

$$E_{e-} = (0.70)(16.98\ MeV) \approx 11.9\ MeV$$

$$E_{e+} = (0.30)(16.98\ MeV) = 5.1\ MeV$$

Worksheet 8-2: Photon Attenuation/Half-Value Layer

I.

1.

$$I = I_o e^{-u_e x}$$

$$= (10^4)\,e^{-(0.58\ cm-1)(3\ cm)}$$

$$= (10^4)\,e^{-1.74}$$

$$= (10^4)(0.1755)$$

2.
$$\approx 1755\ photons\ transmitted$$

$$I = I_o e^{-\mu_1 x}$$

$$\left(1.5\frac{mR}{hr}\right) = \left(200\frac{mR}{hr}\right)e^{-\mu_1 x}$$

$$= e^{-\mu_1 x} = \frac{1.5\frac{mR}{hr}}{200\frac{mR}{Hr}} \approx 0.0075$$

Take ln of both sides and using the rule that ln y^x = x ln y:

$$\ln(e^{-\mu_1 x}) = \ln(0.0075)$$

$$-\mu_1 x(1) = -4.89$$

$$-(0.87\ cm^{-1})(x) = -4.89$$

$$x = \frac{4.89}{0.87\,cm^{-1}} \approx 5.6\ cm\ of\ Pb\ needed$$

3a.

$$I = I_0 e^{-\mu_1 x}$$

$$\frac{I}{I_0} = e^{-\mu_1 x}$$

Note I/I_0 is the fraction of the beam transmitted.

$$I = I_0 e^{-\mu_e x}$$

$$= (10^4) e^{-(0.58 cm^{-1})(3\ cm)}$$

$$= (10^4) e^{-1.74}$$

$$= (10^4)(0.1755)$$

$$\approx 1755\ photons\ transmitted$$

$$\frac{I}{I_0} = e^{-(0.82 cm^{-1})(0.5\ cm)}$$

$$= e^{-0.41}$$

$$\approx 0.66 \quad (thus\ {\sim}66\%\ of\ the\ beam\ will\ be\ transmitted)$$

b. $\%\ attenuation = 100\% - \%\ transmission$

$$= 100\% - 66\%$$

$$\approx 34\%\ attenuated$$

c.
$$HVL = \frac{0.693}{\mu_1}$$

$$= \frac{0.693}{0.82\ cm^{-1}} \approx 0.85\ cm\ of\ steel$$

4a.
$$I = I_0 (0.5)^N$$

$$\frac{I}{I_0} = (0.5)^N = fraction\ transmitted$$

$$= (0.5)^{\frac{3.2mm}{1.2mm}}$$

$$= (0.5)^{2.67}$$

$$\approx 0.157 \quad (thus\ {\sim}15.7\%\ of\ the\ beam\ will\ be\ transmitted)$$

b.

$$\frac{I}{I_0} = (0.5)^N$$

$$= (0.5)^{\frac{2.6mm}{1.2mm}}$$

$$= (0.5)^{2.17}$$

$$= 0.22 \quad (thus \sim 22\% \; is \; transmitted \; and \sim 78\% \; is \; attenuated)$$

5a. 15% attenuated implies 85% is transmitted, therefore

$$\frac{I}{I_0} = (0.5)^N$$

$$(0.85) = (0.5)^N$$

First solve for N:

$$\ln(0.5)^N = \ln(0.85)$$

$$N(-0.693) \approx -0.163$$

$$N \approx \frac{-0.163}{-0.693} \approx 0.23$$

Recall that $N = \dfrac{thickness \; of \; absorber}{HVL}$, *therefore*

$$HVL = \frac{thickness}{N}$$

$$= \frac{1.8mm}{0.23} \approx 7.8mm \; Pb$$

b. 15% of the beam is transmitted, therefore

$$\frac{I}{I_0} = (0.5)^N$$

$$(0.15) = (0.5)^N$$

Solve for N:

$$\ln(0.5)^N = \ln 0.15$$

$$N \ln 0.5 = \ln 0.15$$

$$N(-0.693) \approx 1.897$$

$$N = \frac{-1.897}{-0.693} \approx 2.74$$

Recall that $N = \dfrac{thickness \; of \; absorber}{HVL}$, *then*

$$HVL = \frac{thickness}{N}$$

$$= \frac{1.8mm}{2.74} \approx 0.66mm \; Pb$$

6a.

$$I = I_o(0.5)^N$$

$$\left(0.5 \frac{mR}{hr}\right) = \left(150 \frac{mR}{hr}\right)(0.5)^N$$

$$(0.5)^N = \frac{0.5 \frac{mR}{hr}}{150 \frac{mR}{hr}} \approx 0.0033$$

Solving for N,

$$\ln(0.5)^N = \ln(0.0033)$$

$$N(-0.693) = -5.704$$

$$N = \frac{-5.704}{-0.693} \approx 8.23$$

Recalling $N = \dfrac{thickness\ of\ Absorber}{HVL}$, *then*

$$thickness = (N)(HVL)$$

$$\approx (8.23)(0.2mm\ Pb)$$

$$\approx 1.65\ mm\ Pb\ needed$$

7a. ~ 9.5% transmitted

 b. ~5.4% transmitted, therefore ~94.6% is attenuated

 c. ~2.3 HVLs

Worksheet 10-1: Film

1. b

2. a

3. a

4. a

5. d

6. a

7. a

8. a

9. c

10. c

11. b

12. b

13. b

14. e

15. a

16. d

17. toe

18. speed

19. film constrast

20. shoulder

21. maximum density

Worksheet 15-1: Fluoroscopy

1. c

2. a

3. a

4. a

5. d

6. b

7. a

8. c

9. b

10. a

11. x-rays

12. input phosphor

13. photocathode

14. electrons

15. electrostatic lenses

16. image intensifier tube

17. anode

18. electrons

19. fluorescent screen

20. light photons

Worksheet 16-1: Equipment Malfunctions and Misapplications

1. a. Push bucky tray all the way into table/holder.

   b. Put tube crane in proper position to close SID switch.

   c. Check to make sure only one of the cassette holders (table or upright) is engaged.

2. a. Wrong speed image receptor was used - check and use proper speed.

   b. Cassette is used upside down - use cassette properly.

3. a. Center part correctly.

   b. Use longer back-up time.

   c. Use correct detector chamber.

   d. Set correct density.

4. Notify Quality Control supervisor or service engineer.

5. Hand switch, relay, or bucky may need servicing - contact QC supervisor or service engineer.

Worksheet 17-1:   Quality Control

1. b

2. c

3. d

4. d

5. b

6. c

7. b

8. a

9. a

10. d

11. a

12. d

13. b

14. b (note: a repeat analysis will only provide clues that will require additional analysis to determine cause).

15. a

Worksheet 18-1:   General Radiation Biology

1. b

2. d

3. b

4. a

5. d

6. b

7. b

8. b

9. a

10. c

11. c,b,a,d

12. b

13. Latent period

14. Gastrointestinal syndrome

15. Recovery or death

Worksheet 18-2: General Radiation Biology

1. b

2. a

3. d

4. d

5. c

6. a

7. c

8. c

9. a

10. b

Worksheet 19-1: Applying Radiation Biology to Clinical Practice

1. c

2. a

3. b

4. d

5. c

6. c

7. c

8. c

9. a

10. c

11. c

12. b

3. c

Worksheet 21-1: Radiation Protection

1. c

2. a

3. a

4. b

5. b

6. c

7. b

8. c

9. a

10. b

11. +

12. -

13. +

14. -

15. -